Vibrational Energy
for a little unfair
Career Success

by Gloria Gold

Introduction to Energy Vibration

'There simply is not enough action in the world to compensate for the misalignment of energy, when you care about how you feel and you tend to your vibrational balance first, then you experience what feels like a cooperative universe that seems to open doors everywhere.'

- Abraham

Dearest reader, like so many people in this time, you may find yourself in a career or work environment that brings a massive dose of frustration along with some joy or satisfaction. You may be one of the blessed few, already pursuing or living your dream job. You may, like most people, be slogging through the nine to five just to pay the bills. You might be looking to jump careers, or you might be desperately trying to find any job so that you *can* pay the bills.

Don't you worry for another minute! Wherever you find yourself right now, you will see that by adding the vibration of essential oils, gemstones, and other seemingly magical tools, you *will* increase the joy, satisfaction, and overall fabulousness of your work-life experience.

If you answer yes to any of these questions, then this book can be your guiding light to ease, joy and delight and will give you so many reasons to celebrate.

What you need is a little unfair advantage.

In this book, I share some powerful vibrational tools that will help you to create a seemingly magical shift in your work life. Used with intent, these tools can help you to get your ideal job, get that promotion or that pay increase you know you deserve. They will boost your creativity and workplace joy, and banish office politics. These vibrational tools will give you the confidence to shine in a room full of people, be they your colleagues, your leaders, or hundreds of delegates at a conference.

What is vibrational energy and how can it be used to improve your workplace experience?

'Everything in life is vibration' - Albert Einstein

Everything vibrates. Every single thing, from the things that look solid (like a table), through to the things that we can't even see (like our thoughts), is made up of vibrational energy. Quantum physics is now able to conclusively show us that everything in our universe is energy. This energy vibrates at different frequencies, which then become magnets for energy which is vibrating at a similar rate. Like attracts like.

This Law of Vibration is the basis for the Law of Attraction. Whatever is in someone's life is there because it matches the vibration from their thoughts and their feelings.

So, by aligning with specific vibrational frequencies, you will be able to attract similar energies that will positively impact your work experience.

For this to work, you don't have to understand the science behind this vibrational law of attraction. What is important is that you choose the tools that resonate with you, and that you use them with the right intent. Over the next couple of days and weeks, you will see the enormous impact this has in your life.

In this book I have focused on seven vibrational modalities, being -

Essential oils

Crystals and gemstones

Numbers

Colors

Switchwords

Angels and deities

And sigils.

We'll look at specific elements within these, so that you are well equipped to attract the desired changes into your work experience. Some will resonate more with you, and those will be the best ones for you to work with.

Along with the modalities and elements that have the most aligned vibration to help you address these areas, I have also grouped workplace challenges into broad areas of concern, being -

Getting that promotion

Finding a job

Bringing joy to your job

Boosting creativity

Clearing office politics (including bad boss vibes)

And speaking in public

At the end of each workplace challenge section, you can create an energy circle. The energy circle charges and empowers the elements that you've chosen to work with, so that you can get the greatest benefit from the vibrational magnet that you are creating.

While I cannot promise that you will instantly become the CEO of your company, earning a seven-figure salary, these tools have stood the test of time. When used with the right intent they will lift the burden of work, and will create more joy, more success, and much more of what you want in your career.

Using the Table of Contents, you can go directly to the specific workplace challenge that you need to address, or you can read through from start to finish. Part One covers a broad description of each modality and explains how to use that modality, and Part Two gives your tools for each of the workplace challenges. As you read, note the elements that resonate with you.

The sooner you begin, the sooner you will experience a GOLDEN SUNRISE in your career, so let's get going now.

PART ONE

VIBRATIONAL MODALITIES

Essential Oils

What are Essential Oils

Essential oils are highly concentrated oils extracted from plant material. These are extracted by varying methods, like steam distillation, and cold-pressing. Generally it is the most aromatic part of the plant that is used, for example, rose oil is extracted from the rose petals, while black pepper oil is made from the berries, or peppercorns, of the Piperaceae plant.

How to use Essential Oils

Essential oils can be up to 75 times more potent than dried herbs, and carry strong, energetic vibrations of both their individual components and of the whole plant. Some oils can be applied neat to your skin. I do recommend that you add your essential oil to a carrier oil like Sweet Almond oil, Jojoba oil, Grape Seed oil or Coconut oil before applying it. Essential oils can evaporate quite quickly, and a carrier oil helps the effects to last that much longer. You can add essential oils to your bath water or a water-based spritzer. Great for office clearing and lifting everyone's mood, is to add your essential oil mix to a diffuser allowing the oils to weave their magic throughout the office.

It is essential to do a sensitivity test before using any oil extensively. The best way to do this is to mix two drops of neat oil with half a teaspoon of carrier oil. Apply this mixture onto the inner crease of your elbow, and watch if you have any reaction over the next 24 hours.

Using the right essential oils can almost instantly raise your vibration to be a match to the desired state that you're after.

Here are just a few examples of oils that can help you feel calmer, more energized, increase your confidence and some oils that will put you in a good mood.

Oils for confidence - Bergamot, Cedarwood, Coriander, Jasmine Absolute

Oils for physical energy - The citrus oils like Sweet Orange and Lemon, Peppermint, Cinnamon

Uplifting Oils - Neroli, Basil, Peppermint, Frankincense, Cedarwood, Juniper

Calming Oils - Lavender, Roman Chamomile, Rose

Crystals and Gemstones

What are crystals and gemstones

Crystals and Gemstones are one of the most stable sources of vibration for all types of energy work, and have been used by most major traditions over thousands of years.

Crystals form over time; as liquids in the earth begin to solidify, common molecules and ions draw together to become more stable, in a uniform and repeating pattern, which creates the crystal. Some crystals, like diamonds, are formed under high pressure in carbon. Natural crystals have been growing inside the Earth's crust for over a million years. These crystals and gemstones have specific high vibrational frequencies and have the power to serve you across a wide range of needs. From clearing negative energy to physical healing, spiritual attunement, and all-round raising vibrations, crystals help you to align with your desired state.

Healing Benefits of Crystals and Gemstones

Crystals and gemstones emit positive, uplifting, energizing, and calming vibrations. Working with crystals and gemstones will help you achieve a more peaceful mind and a revitalized physical state of being. Holding crystals, placing them on your body or in your environment can promote physical, emotional, mental, and spiritual healing.

Some crystals alleviate stress and improve mood; others improve concentration or creativity; some are calming, while others are energizing and stimulating. There is probably a crystal for every need that you have.

Different crystals have their own vibration powers or energy

Here are some examples of crystals that can heal, raise your vibration to attract love, prosperity, to keep you safe and protected, and more.

Clear quart - This crystal is a "master healer." Clear quartz absorbs, clears, and releases stuck energy. Clear quartz improves concentration and memory. Clear quartz can stimulate the immune system and bring the body back into balance. This stone is often paired with other quartz crystals to enhance their qualities. It strengthens intentions; helps to clear and open the chakras; increases psychic visions, spiritual development, and growth; improves clarity, concentration, and harmony.

Rose quartz - This gentle pink stone is also called the 'love' stone, improving all relationships, and creating deeper connections. Rose quartz also provides comfort during times of grief. Rose quartz encourages love, respect, trust, and self-worth.

Jasper - This loving stone is known as the "supreme nurturer." Jasper supports you in stressful times by giving you the courage to face the challenges. It absorbs negative energy and builds courage, quick thinking, and confidence. These qualities are helpful when tackling painful issues — which is precisely where this stone can assist.

Citrine - This orangy yellow quartz brings positivity and enthusiasm to every part of your life. Citrine clears stuck energy and negativity and encourages optimism, warmth, motivation, and clarity. It enhances mindful qualities like creativity and concentration.

Turquoise - This bright blue crystal has powers that can help to heal the mind, body, and soul. Turquoise is used as a good luck charm that can help balance your emotions. Physically, turquoise benefits the respiratory, skeletal, and immune system.

Tiger's eye. This golden-hued crystal clears fear, anxiety, and self-doubt. Tiger's eye guides you to harmony and balance and helps you to make clear, conscious decisions.

Black Onyx - This shiny black stone is a powerful protection stone that absorbs and transforms negative energy. Black onyx helps you build emotional and physical strength, especially when you need support in times of stress, confusion, or grief.

Cleaning and charging your crystals

When you first receive your gems, they may have absorbed energies from the previous owner or the store. It's best to clear the crystal from these energies. You will also need to cleanse your crystals regularly as you work with them, and they absorb energies from you and your environment.

How to clean your crystals and gemstones

Use any of the methods below that best resonates with you. Don't soak your softer or more crumbly crystals in water as they can disintegrate a bit.

- Hold your gemstones under running water for a few minutes..
- Soak them soaked overnight in a saltwater solution or seawater.
- Cover them in uncooked brown rice which absorbs the old energy - remember to throw out or bury the brown rice after three months of regular use.
- Crystals can also be cleared and charged on a large crystal cluster if you have one.

Once cleared, it is good to charge the crystals either by sunlight, moonlight, or a combination of both.

You can also programme your crystal with your specific intention. Sit in a calm, meditative state. Hold your crystal and be open to feeling it's specific frequency. When you have a sense of this, you can then let the crystal know exactly what vibrational energy you need from it. As an example, 'I need you to vibrate at the level of confidence and vitality for me'. Once you feel that you have communicated your needs, you can thank the crystal, and send it love.

Angels and Deities

The vibrational power Angels

Angels are spiritual beings; said to be the messengers between God and humans. Angels are constantly at a high vibration, and so come with great love and non-judgement.

You can tap into the divine power of angels to support your needs or change any negative energy around you through meditation, affirmations, and prayer.

Here are some examples

For financial prosperity, you can call on Archangel Ariel.

'Dearest Archangel Ariel, I call you on you now. Please help me to release all blocks that are stopping me from receiving the abundance that is always flowing towards me. Help me to feel worthy of receiving this abundance. Thank you, thank you, thank you.'

When you are confused or are struggling to make the right choice, pray to Archangel Jeremiel.

'Dear Archangel Jeremiel, please help me to release the fear and misinformation that is clouding my mind. So that I can clearly see the right way forward, in service of the highest good of all concerned. Thank you!'

When in need of protection, courage, and strength, pray to Archangel Michael.

"Archangel Michael, I call on you now. I ask that you place your deep blue cloak of protection over me, keeping me safe and protected, now and always. Thank you, thank you, thank you.'

The vibrational power of Deities

The word deity means a "divine being." Deities are also called gods and goddesses, and are supernatural beings with specific qualities and gifts. Most ancient cultures prayed to deities that they attributed certain qualities to, often times to better understand the natural world around them, like thunderstorms, droughts, good harvest etc.

Examples of Deities from various cultures

Greek deities - they include Zeus, Hera Poseidon Ares Hephaestus Athena Hermes Demeter, Aphrodite, Dionysus, Artemis, Apollo, Hestia, Hades, Persephone, Hercules.

Hindu deities - they include Ganesh, Elephant-headed god, Kali, Trimurti/Triumvirate, Brahma, Vishnu, Shiva, Krishna, Saraswati, Lakshmi, Durga, Satyanarayana, Rama.

Egyptian - Ra, Horus, Anubis, Aken, Anhur, Aker, Ammit, Amunet, Onuris, Sobek, Shu, Tatenen, Taweret.

You can change your vibration by aligning with the energy of a deity through mantra, prayer, and meditation.

Here are examples of deities and their vibrational energy

For wealth, pray to Lakshmi, the Hindu goddess of wealth and prosperity.

'Om Shreem Maha Lakshmiyei Namaha' It is best to repeat this mantra, and other Hindu deity mantras, 108 times each day, for 33 or 40 days, in a calm, meditative state.

For courage and wisdom, call on the Greek goddess Athena.

'I call on Goddess Athena, goddess of courage and wisdom. Give me strength and courage to face my darkness, which now comes in the physical form of (name the challenge). Help me to heal this low vibrational aspect of myself, so that my world reflects my joy and peace.'

Call on the Buddhist and Tibetan deity Tara for relief and protection from the eight fears. These fears are outer physical dangers, and the inner dangers of ignorance, attachment, anger, pride, jealousy, miserliness, doubt and wrong views.

'Om Tare Tuttare Ture So Ha'. It is best to repeat this mantra, and other Buddhist mantras, 108 times, as many times as necessary.

Vibrational Power of Numbers

What is numerology

Numerology is how we simplify sacred math and how we apply it to understand aspects of our existence. Our love life, career, health, family life, friendships, spirituality, leisurely activities, and personality can all be mathematically explained and understood through the study of numbers and their vibration.

According to Balliett and modern numerologists, each number has a specific vibration. The numbers one to nine have unique properties that are the direct result of their inherent vibration. To determine a person's number, the numerologist adds the individual numbers in their date of birth. If the answer has more than a single number, these individual numbers are again added, to arrive at a single-digit number, unless the double figures are 11, 22 or 33. These are Master numbers and carry a high vibration.

For example: If you were born on 31 07 1998. Add all the single numbers together - 3+1+0+7+1+9+9+8=38. If this is not a single number, or a master number, continue to add these single numbers together - 3+8=11. This is a master number, so no need to distil it further to a 2.

The various types of Numerology

Kabbalah Numerology. It originated from Hebrew mysticism based on the Hebrew alphabet. It has only 22 vibrations because of the different alphabet. Kabbalah, which means knowledge that comes through the mind and soul, interprets the meaning of names. It is also called Name Numerology.

Chaldean Numerology. Chaldean Numerology assigns each letter with a number based on the letter's vibration, rather than following the alphabetical order. Chaldean numerology analyzes both name and date of birth.

1	2	3	4	5	6	7	8
A	B	C	D	E	U	O	F
I	K	G	M	H	V	Z	P
J	R	L	T	N	W		
O		S		X			

Pythagorean Numerology. Generally used in modern-day numerology and was created by the Greek philosopher Pythagoras. Pythagorean numerology looks at the interaction between the name and date of birth. The letters of the alphabet are assigned numbers in their alphabetical order, using the numbers 1 through 9.

1	2	3	4	5	6	7	8	9
A	B	C	D	E	F	G	H	I
J	K	L	M	N	O	P	Q	R
S	T	U	V	W	X	Y	Z	

The vibrational energy of each number

Number 1 resonates with pioneering, beginnings, individuation, raw power, force, activity, leadership, courage, truth, assertiveness, initiative, instinct, and intuition.

Number 2 is the vibration and energy of balance, peace, diplomacy, intuition, emotion, unions, love and sensitivity.

Number 3 resonates with the energy of optimism and joy, inspiration and creativity, speech and communication, good taste, imagination and intelligence, sociability and society, friendliness, kindness, and compassion.

Number 4 is practical, organized, and precise. Service, patience, devotion, trust, and building solid foundations are substantial number four energies.

Number 5 is a free, non-attached individual. Five can create change, life lessons learned through experience, and is adaptable and versatile. Five has strong social energy.

Number 6 is the vibration of nurturing, caring, and harmony. They also say that it's a sexy six.

Number 7 resonates with the vibrations and energies of the collective consciousness, faith, and spirituality, spiritual awakening, and awareness, spiritual enlightenment, spiritual development.

Number 8 vibrates with authority and personal power, self-confidence, confidence, inner-strength, professionalism, success, good judgment, and abundance.

Number 9 vibrates with childlike wonder, having completed the egoic cycle, the nine can return to playfulness, creative abilities, brilliance, inner-wisdom, self-love, freedom, high ideals, tolerance, humility, altruism, and benevolence.

Master Numbers

Double or triple numbers made up of the same digit are known as master numbers; these are a higher vibration due to this pairing.

Master Number 11 combines the double masculine energy of the one with the feminine energy of the two. This combination creates a shade and light, heaven and earth merging, bringing a higher vibrational energy.

Master Number 22, also known as the Master Builder, is the second master number, bringing deep spiritual understanding. This double impact of the feminine two, along with the stability and foundational elements of the four brings the vibrational essence of the 11 into physical expression.

Master Number 33. This master number combines the double energy of three, expression, with the teacher/caregiver energy of the six, to take the 11 and 22 into enlightenment as the Master Teacher and the most spiritually evolved of all numbers.

Light and Color Energy

We see light in the form of color. Each wavelength and frequency within the visible light spectrum is seen as a different color, bringing its unique energetic resonance. Even though the color spectrum is continuous, we group visible light into the seven colors, as reflected in the rainbow, and our chakras, or energy centers - Red, Orange, Yellow, Green, Blue, Indigo, and Violet.

By understanding how the vibration of each color influences us, we can use color to support us in many different ways.

Colors and their vibrational energies.

An easy way to help create your desired reality is through using colors that align with the vibrations of what you want. For example, you can wear the color in your clothing or jewelry; you can keep a little piece of paper or fabric in that color in your pocket or purse; you can use that colored pen for making notes; your device screens can have that color as the background and screensaver.

Here is a list of colors and their vibrations

Red - The color of fire, blood, and the red earth. Red is the vibration of leadership, unity, focused concentration, and action. Red also exhibits vitality, courage, self-confidence. Red is passion, passionate love, or heated argument. Red stimulates the appetite, increases blood pressure, and speeds up metabolism. Red is the color of the root chakra.

Orange - The blend of red and yellow. Orange encourages cooperation, balance, and harmony of inner worlds and outer environments. This color will support you in learning, bringing peace to relationships, increasing your happiness and success. Orange increases oxygen supply to the brain and invigorates us. Orange brings joy and life to the environment; it helps us to connect with others and brings the introvert out to play. Orange is the color of the sacral chakra.

Yellow - The color of sunshine. The vibration of communication, optimism, joy, and self-expression. This color will support you in stimulating creativity and confidence. Yellow increases our ability to perceive and understand by connecting to our mental self. Yellow is the color of the solar plexus chakra.

Green - The color of nature. The vibration of growth, harmony, freshness, and fertility. This color will support you in cultivating inner peace, relaxation, responsibility, growth, abundance, and prosperity. Green is excellent for improving eyesight. The color of the heart chakra.

Blue - The color of the sky and the oceans. The vibration of trust, loyalty, wisdom, confidence, intelligence, faith, truth, and heaven. Blue suppresses the appetite. Blue relaxes our mind; it calms the nervous system and helps us to relax. Ideal for sleep problems and hyperactive children. Blue is the color of the throat chakra.

Indigo - The vibration of nurturing, intuition, and beauty. Indigo shifts us past the separation of our egoic selves, allowing us to see ourselves as part of the whole. Indigo is the color of the third eye chakra.

Violet - The vibration of spirituality, knowledge, and wisdom. Because of its high vibration, violet can transmute lower frequencies into its own.

You can call on the gold, silver and violet flame of harmony and transmutation, to shift lower energies into high vibration energy.

Switchwords

Sigmund Freud first noted Switchwords. He found that certain words have the power to bypass our conscious mind, and reach directly into our subconscious. James T. Mangan, whose book, The Secret of Perfect Living, was the first person to cover information about the power of switchwords in greater detail.

What are Switchwords?

Switchwords are everyday words that have a direct impact on the subconscious. This vibrational impact may or may not be related to the actual meaning of the word in the way we use it in our language. The switchword BLUFF can be used to reduce anxiety, which is very far from its English meaning. The switchword SHINE helps you to improve your mood quickly, likened to sunshine.

How to Use Switchwords

The full list of switchwords is extensive. It is possible to create a switchword phrase (SWP) linking more than one switchword to boost the power of your new 'mantra.' Less is more. It is more effective to stick to one or two switchwords rather than stringing a whole lot together, as they may nullify each other's vibrations.

Once you have found the best switchword for your needs or created a suitable switchword phrase, you can repeat it as often as you remember, or when that issue comes up. There is a school of thought that suggests that you repeat your SWP either 28 or 108 times twice a day.

It is more powerful to write the switchword out or to say it out loud, and less compelling to say it in your mind. When writing switchwords, use CAPITAL letters.

Power switchwords

These switchwords can be added to more instructional switchwords to give them an added boost.

TOGETHER - this switchword aligns your conscious and subconscious so that both minds focus on the same intended outcome.

DIVINE - this switchword vibrates at the highest level, blessing the switchword phrase.

GOLDEN SUNRISE is another powerful SWP which lifts the instructional switchword to a whole new vibration.

Sigils

What is a Sigil

The word sigil comes from the Latin word sigillum, meaning seal. Historically sigil was used to refer to a coat of arms or an identifying sign generally. Often sigils would consist of a figure of something which would represent their family. Sometimes these sigils were accompanied by inscriptions, like the family motto. A sigil is also an inscribed or painted symbol considered to have magical power. In medieval times, magicians would summon powerful beings through the symbol or sigil created from their names.

In modern usage, a sigil is a simple but powerful symbol that we create to bypass the conscious mind and directly impact the subconscious mind with our desired outcome.

How to create a sigil

The simplest way to create a desire sigil is to write out your desired state in a short positive statement. For example, if you wanted to lose some weight, your statement could be - I AM SLIM, VITAL, VIBRANT AND HEALTHY

From the initial statement, you then remove all vowels, just keeping the consonants - MSLMVTLVBRNTNDHLTHY

From here, remove any duplicate letters - MSLVTBRNDHY

Using just these remaining letters, draw a symbol. It may take several iterations to get a design that you like, and the result can enjoy some creative license.

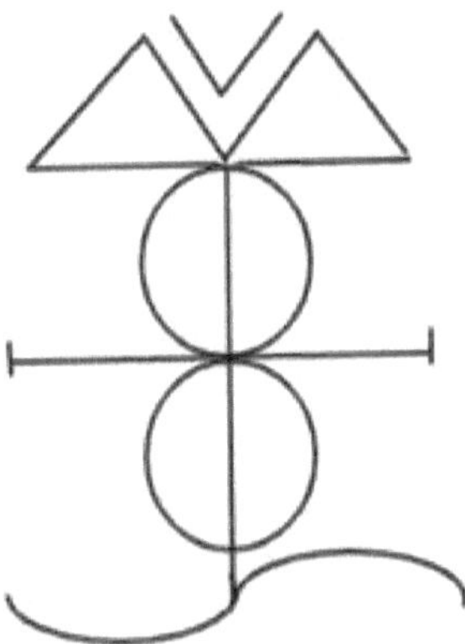

You can then place this sigil wherever it will most impact your desired outcome, in this instance, on the fridge door, on your bathroom mirror, etc.

Types of Sigils

The main uses/types of sigils are covered below.

Desire Sigil

As used in the example above, a desire sigil is a sigil focused around a desired state that you wish to manifest. You can use desire sigils for anything that you want to bring forward. It could be an abundance sigil, a sigil for love, even a sigil to have a successful job interview. The energetic vibration of the sigil bypasses your logical mind, to directly impact your subconscious.

Name Sigil

You can create your name sigil that you can include when asking for something you desire. Create a name sigil for the car brand that you wish to own, right through to a quality that you want to vibrate at, like a deity or Angel's name.

Correspondence Sigil

Correspondence sigils are symbolic representations of aspects that you wish to work with, but can't access. For example, you could create the correspondence sigil of money if you want to include that aspect in your energy circle.

Energy Circles

What is an energy circle

An energy circle is a focused gathering of all the elements that you have selected to achieve your desired outcome. Write your full name, and place each of the items chosen inside a drawn energy circle. The energy circle gathers and concentrates the vibrational effects of each of the elements, adding power to your intentions.

How to create an energy circle

Start building your energy circle by writing your name at the top center of the page in the area that you will circle.

Write a concise phrase about what you intend to manifest.

Then add switchwords, deities and angels, crystals (either just write the name of the crystal or actually place the crystal in your circle), essential oils (again, either write the name, place the bottle or add a few drops of the oil into your energy circle), numbers, colours, your sigil and anything else that will boost your intention.

Then draw a complete circle around everything that you have placed on the page. The circle should close neatly and should not touch any of the elements within the circle. It should be one continuous circular line with no interruptions.

Energy Circles work best when in an open space so that their vibration can extend outwards. Keeping your circle in a closed book stops it's vibration entirely.

Once you have achieved the desired outcome, you can tear up the energy circle and release the focused energy.

Knowing which elements will work best for you

We will be covering a number of elements, and each one could seem more magnificent than the other, leaving you confused as to which ones will work best for you, or it could make you want to use all of them which achieves cluttered and diluted results. There are several ways that you can select the specific items within each modality to get the best results for your particular needs.

Intellect

You can read about each of the elements, and based on the descriptions; you can make your mind up.

Gut feel

Sometimes it's more powerful to bypass the logic of your mind and to trust your gut. Gut feelings are often the culmination of past experiences and subtle nuances that the conscious mind cannot access. Using gut feel, you would select a particular element if it excites you when reading its name or its properties. I often know which element is right for me because I get a slight thrill in my gut when reading about that element. Trust your gut.

Pendulum

Using a pendulum to help you make your selection can also be very effective. If you don't have a pendulum, you can use a necklace chain/cord with a weight hanging from it, like a ring, or a pendant. The cord and weight should be able to swing freely when held between two fingers.

The first step is to determine your 'yes' and your 'no' when using a pendulum. Pendulums tend to swing in three directions, it could swing in a circle to the right, it could rotate to the left, or it could swing in a straight line up and down. You can check with your real name by saying, 'My name is (and your actual name)' and see how the pendulum swings. That would be your 'yes'. Counter check this by saying, 'My name is (and another name, not your own) and see how the pendulum swings. That would be your 'no'. You can test this several times to be sure. The pendulum may swing right for 'yes' and left for 'no'; it may swing up and down for one of the answers etc. Once you have a clear signal of what is your 'yes' and what is your 'no,' you can then use your pendulum to help you select your elements.

First, check with your pendulum by asking permission, for example - 'Can you tell me which elements will best help me to achieve my specific objective?'. If you get a 'yes' signal, then you can continue.

Holding your pendulum in one hand, use your other hand to point out each element one at a time. For each one, note whether the pendulum gives a 'yes' or 'no' signal. Once you have the list of elements that will work best for you, your 'yes' elements, you can double-check with the pendulum saying, 'Are these the best elements to help me with my specific desire?' If too many are selected, you can go through the process again, telling the pendulum that you only want the top three elements, as an example.

Muscle testing

Muscle testing is another effective way to bypass the logic mind. There are several methods that you can use, with a weak muscle response meaning 'no' and a strong muscle response indicating 'yes'.

One approach is to hold your arm out in front of you, parallel to the ground. Use your other hand to push down on the straight arm when asking a question. Use the name question described in the pendulum section above to test whether this method will work well for you. If the raised arm remains firm with your real name and easy to press down with your false name, you can use muscle testing for an effective yes and no response.

Another way to use muscle testing is to make a closed circle with your thumb and forefinger. You can then attempt to push your other hand through this circle to test for a yes or no. If the ring holds firm its a yes if the circle easily gives way its a no. Muscle testing may work better if you have a friend testing your muscle strength so that the consistency of force remains unbiased.

Clarifying your request

The more single-minded and focused you are about your desired outcome, the more easily it can come to you. Your vibration dilutes when your thoughts are concentrated in one direction today, and a different direction tomorrow. You will begin attracting a different thing each day, and so nothing much comes to pass.

At the beginning of each workplace challenge, I ask some questions that you can use to help clarify what it is that you desire. Your answers will help you to be very clear about where you are directing both your energy, and the vibration of the energy tools that you are using. Things speed up when everything is working towards the same outcome.

Dearest reader, if you find value in this book, I would SO appreciate a review on Amazon Kindle, so that my book can reach and impact more readers. Here's the link: https://www.amazon.com/kindle/dp/B07ZMZDR5Q/ref=r dr_kindle_ext_eos_detail

PART TWO

VIBRATIONAL TOOLS FOR CAREER SUCCESS

Vibrational Energy to draw in a Promotion

Vibrational energy can boost your chance of getting that promotion by

Boosting your confidence

Improving your leadership vibration

Increasing your positivity

Improving your persuasive abilities For help during the interview)

Raising your vibration of power and more.

Clarifying your request

What will your new title be?

What are the key responsibilities of this role?

How much do you expect to earn?

Will you manage a team?

If so, how many people will be in your team?

What style of leadership will you have?

What is the physical proof of your promotion - a new parking bay, a bigger office?

What other perks will you receive from this promotion?

Is there anything else that will help you to be really clear about your desire?

If any of these answers make you feel uncomfortable, work through that, or adjust the question and your response, until you have an unmistakable, joyful feeling when you think about receiving this promotion.

Write your clear desire down, and you can add, 'this or better now comes to me.'

Use this statement and joyful feeling when selecting and working with the energy tools that follow.

Essential Oils to draw in a promotion

Cedarwood - This warm and comforting oil can be used for confidence, strength increased power.

Jasmine Absolute - A highly concentrated oil, use just a few drops of this exotic scented oil to boost your confidence.

Laurel (Bay Laurel) - Use the sweet, fruity scent to feel motivated, and to gain energy and strength.

Rosemary - This herbaceous, camphor scented oil instills confidence when filled with self-doubt and improves motivation when faced with challenges.

Calamus - If you want to influence someone to act positively on your behalf, rub a few drops of Calamus on your palms and touch the person.

Camphor - This medicinally smelling oil increases your personal influence and persuasiveness.

Citronella - Well known for its ability to keep mosquitos at bay, citronella also promotes persuasiveness and eloquence.

Basil - This herby, liquorice-like scent can increase business success, happiness and prosperity. It is stimulating so don't use late at night, or you'll be up for a while. Basil has a dominating scent, so use sparingly and blend with other oils, or you may spend the day smelling like basil pesto!

Bergamot - This floral-citrus scented oil is great for business success, physical energy, and increasing prosperity. Bergamot oil is phototoxic, meaning that it can irritate your skin if you are in the sun for too long, giving you 'sunburn' and dark spots, so only use when you won't be in the sun.

Cinnamon - This strongly scented, spicy oil is said to have magical powers. Use it to increase your business success, increase your luck and is very good at bringing in money. This use must be well diluted in a carrier oil before using on your skin, and is better to use in a diffuser.

Ginger Root - This spicy, uplifting oil is a powerful at speeding up your manifestation, it brings progress on all levels. Ginger root oil gives you courage and fire in your belly.

Cardamom - This spicy-woody scented oil awakens a dull mind and dispels tensions and worries during challenging times. If you chew on some cardamom pods before your interview it can also increase your charm.

Peppermint - This strong scented oil works like a power boost for a fatigued mind, making it more sharp and alert.

Lemon - Lemon oil with it's sharp citrus scent dispels confusion and brings clarity of thought.

Grapefruit - Its positive and upbeat scent is the perfect antidote for tension, frustration, irritability, and moodiness.

Crystals and Gemstones to draw in a promotion

Gold Stone – Although this is a manufactured, rather than a natural stone, Goldstone is great help in securing a promotion and advancing your career. It will also help you achieve good fortune. The glittery specks of gold vibration align with success, wealth, and abundance.

Citrine - You can also increase your chances of promotion and a bigger salary using citrine. Keep citrine close to your body and in your workspace. Keep a piece of citrine under your pillow or in your wallet. It can help to attract your ideal job and will have you accepting that promotion before you know it.

Green Aventurine - Keep a piece of green aventurine in your pocket and a second one on your desk at work to boost your leadership skills. Green Aventurine is known as the 'Stone of Opportunity' and brings exceptional luck, especially in attracting wealth and abundance. It can improve your chances of being promoted. Green Aventurine helps to line up all the conditions needed for your success. It helps you to release beliefs and attitudes that could lower your vibration and limit what you attract. Green Aventurine also strengthens your decision-making skills and amplifies leadership qualities. It boosts your charisma and gives you a sense of humor and openness to the ideas of others.

Bloodstone fills you with courage, self-esteem, energy, and protection so that you can embrace all opportunities that come your way. With this light, upbeat energy, you will be able to make the most from each opportunity presented to you.

Numbers to draw in a promotion

Number One - Brings out your leadership ability, strengthens your charisma as a leader, and builds trust in your skills. Working with the vibration of number one, you can become an inspiring and inspired leader. Number one will help you to be creative, confident, efficient, and determined.

Number Twenty-Two - This master number carries the Master Builder vibration. By tapping into this high vibrating energy, you can draw in the opportunity to become the successful leader of a large business. Number 22 can help you to be goal-oriented, and to bring grand visions into reality.

Number Fifteen - This number helps you to release old beliefs and restrictions so that you can draw the new into your life. 15 also represents leadership and will help you to work on your dreams and ambitions.

Colors to draw in a promotion

Gold is the higher vibration of yellow; it brings confidence, business, and financial success. Gold gives you inner strength and helps you to know where your strengths lie. Hang gold fabric in the doorways of your home to draw money in, and light a gold candle for business success. To increase your chances of promotion, wear gold jewelry to work, or keep something gold in your pocket.

Purple is the color associated with royalty. It is a great color to draw in leadership qualities and to be seen as an authority in your field. If you feel that you will be questioned in a meeting, be sure to wear something purple. Purple is the combination of red and blue, bringing in the leadership and passion of red, combined with the authority and knowledge of blue, creating a master vibration.

Green - This nature color promotes prosperity, abundance, and success. Green is especially useful for leadership positions in philanthropic fields, as green carries the energy of the heart.

Red is the color of will and passion. Wear red if you feel that you need to come across as more goal-oriented and dominant.

Angels and Deities to draw in a promotion

Artemis - As the Greek goddess of hunting, she helps you to pursue your career goals with passion and focus.

Nike - Nike is the Greek goddess of victory. She helps you claim your victories and brings success.

Lakshmi - She is the Hindu goddess of good fortune and beauty. Lakshmi will bless you with career success and abundance.

Dana - Dana is an ancient Celtic goddess. Dana instills the energy of leadership within you.

Ganesha - The pot-bellied elephant god Ganesha is the lord of success, knowledge, and wealth. Ganesha clears all obstacles to success.

Chant the Ganesha mantra 108 times each day for 33 days, to clear all obstacles on your path to success - 'Om Gam Ganapataye Namaha'

Switch Words to draw in a promotion

TAKE ON - Leadership and ambition

BREAKTHROUGH - Helps to achieve success. Used to release hurdles. Helps to propel forward in a particular activity.

HERO - Attracts achievement and success. Can make you a role model for all.

GET - Use to attract success, achievements, understanding, and knowledge.

SOPHISTICATE - Increases your fame and helps you to become a leader with style. Excellent for leadership positions in media and fashion.

STAR - Guides your path to success, improves work performance and attracts appreciation from your boss.

TRIUMPH - Brings a successful outcome to any activity. Helps you to come out as the winner.

TRUMP - Success over opponents, critics, and competitors.

VICTORY - gives you the confidence and courage to move quickly towards your goals

UP, PRAISE - Confidence and self-esteem

CLAP - Gets attention and recognition for your work.

CLIMB - Helps to shine more. It is used to move up step by step. Helps to get a new position.

JEWEL - Raises your vibration to a place where you feel secure, confident, and a leader already — strong positivity for success.

KEY - Raise your power and importance, be seen as an authority figure.

SKY - Helps you to shine at work, to push beyond old limits and to come out as a winner.

SOAR - Quickly gets you to a higher position, and to easily remain there.

SUBLIME - Helps to get a promotion by achieving exceptional performance in any field. Lifts emotions and intellect to achieve success.

TAKE - Helps to be a responsible leader. Helps you to receive good things in life. Gives you the power to get and control any situation.

MASCOT - Helps to lead and guide a team. This switchword builds team spirit. Be appreciated and admired as a leader that brings the best out in the group.

Booster Switch Words

DIVINE MAGIC BEGIN NOW - With this switch word phrase (SWP), we surrender to Divine powers. We ask them to begin their magic to fulfill our wishes and to manifest our desires with the Divine grace, love, and care. Use this SWP for any desire.

GOLDEN SUNRISE BRING MAGIC - This switch word phrase calls GOLDEN SUNRISE to bless us with a divine and magical life. It can change our destiny and to clear karma. Chant this SWP while you connect with your goal to draw it in more quickly.

ADD - This master switchword brings more power and strength to whatever you focus on, and helps to promote anything.

SPEED - Quickens the manifestation of abundance and success

CHEERS - increases happiness, joy, good luck, and success. Especially useful for the positive outcome of any event.

AIM - Helps to keep you focused on the goal for a successful outcome.

Creating a Sigil to draw in a promotion

To begin creating your sigil, write out a positive statement that reflects your specific desire. It should be in the present tense, so starting with I AM helps. It should only use positive words. Remember, you can use the sigil that I have created below, but it would be far more powerful for you to create your sigil. Creating your sigil weaves your focused intention into the sigil, making the sigil send a direct message of your intent to your subconscious.

An example would be -

I AM PROMOTED TO MY IDEAL JOB

Remove all vowels

MPRMTDTMYDLJB

Remove any duplicated letters

MPRTDYLJB

Draw a sigil using the shapes of the remaining letters. Below is an example of a sigil using the above phrase. You can use this sigil, either as it is, or as inspiration. Remembering that it is so much more powerful for you to create your own sigil.

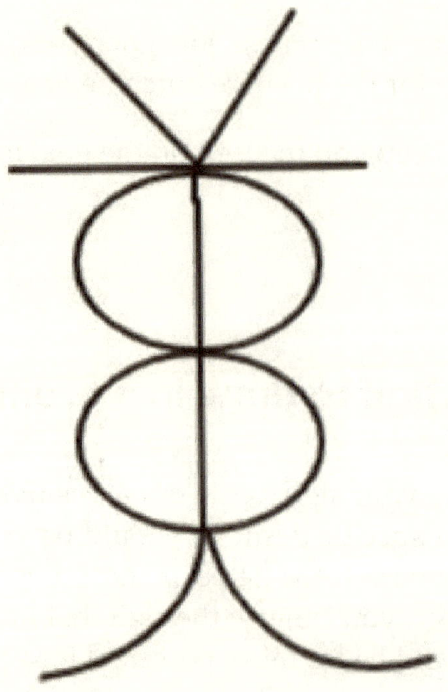

Creating your Energy Circle to draw in promotion

Here is an example of an Energy Circle created to attract a Promotion.

I would also add a drop of basil to my energy circle.

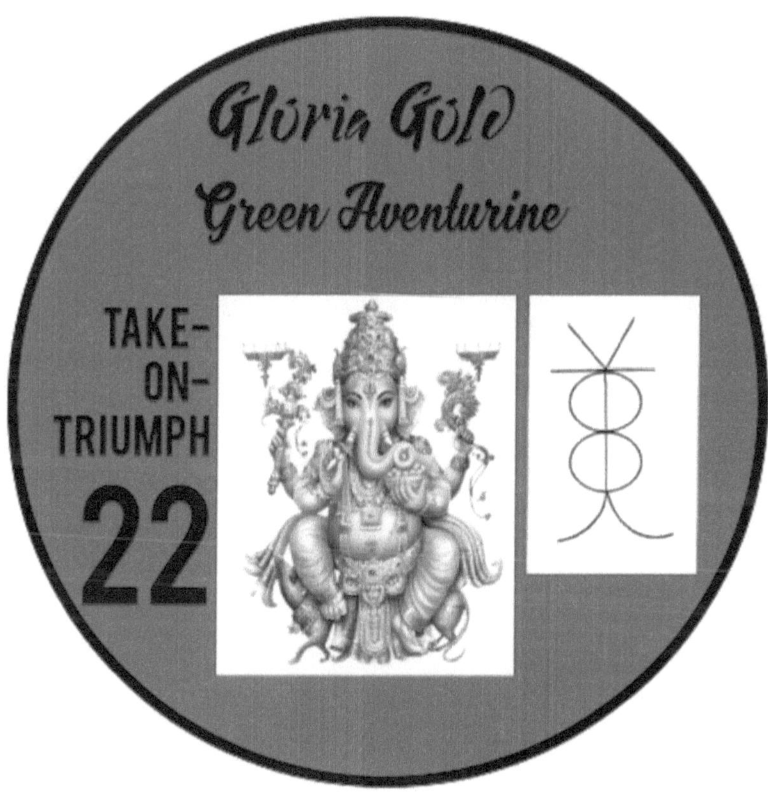

Vibrational Energy to find a New Job

Finding a new job can feel daunting. Vibrational energy can help you by attracting the best job for you, building your confidence, making you more comfortable with change, increasing your luck potential, releasing fears and worries, creating a vibration of abundance and so much more.

Clarifying your request

What will your new title be?

What are the key responsibilities of this role?

How much will you earn?

Will you manage a team?

If so, how many people will be in your team?

Where (which city) will your new job be based?

How far will this job be from your home?

Can you describe the type of company that you want to work for?

Will you need to learn new skills, if so, which skills?

Is there anything else that will help you to clarify what job you want to draw in?

If any of these answers make you feel uncomfortable, work through that, or adjust the question and your response, until you have an unmistakable, joyful feeling when you think about receiving this promotion.

Write your clear desire down, and you can add, 'this or better now comes to me.'

Use this statement and joyful feeling when selecting and working with the energy tools that follow.

Essential oils for finding a new job

Laurel (Bay Laurel) - Use the sweet, fruity scent to feel motivated, and to gain energy and strength.

Rosemary - This herbaceous, camphor scented oil instills confidence when filled with self-doubt and improves motivation when faced with challenges.

Calamus - If you want to influence someone to act positively on your behalf, rub a few drops of Calamus on your palms and touch the person.

Camphor - This medicinally smelling oil increases your personal influence and persuasiveness.

Ylang Ylang - This heady, sweet scented oil is especially powerful in helping you to find a job. Be sure to wear Ylang Ylang to the interview to help you appear calm and confident.

All Spice (Pimento Berry) - This sharp, spicy scent is very energizing, and will boost your spirits if job hunting is wearing you down. This oil can be sensitive to skins, dilute weo

Essential Oils for de-stressing include rose, clary sage, frankincense, lavender, bergamot, marjoram, ylang-ylang, lemon, geranium, orange, sandalwood, chamomile, and vetiver.

Also, see Essential Oils for Getting that Promotion which can help you to draw success towards your job searching endeavors.

Crystals for finding a good job

Jade - This beautiful gem brings good luck. Jade opens you up to receive prosperity and abundance. Tapping into ancient wisdom, Jade can help you see your challenges from a much broader perspective. Jade brings a sense of peace which allows you to see through stress and tension to have a clear vision of who you can be.

Garnet - Garnet brings success and achievement. It also dispels panic, worry, and fears. Wear garnet to feel grounded and secure, knowing that you will be supported. Garnet brings light and hope and increases self-confidence.

Sodalite - This vibrant blue stone improves your sense of self-worth, self-esteem, and self-acceptance. It helps you to move from an overly emotional state to a more logical state, great for interviews. Sodalite improves your will and determination and reduces anxiety and panic.

Malachite - This "stone of transformation" gives you confidence, good fortune, and abundance. Malachite can transform a vibration of lack into one of success. It can bring lucrative offers to you. Malachite boosts confidence and releases any sense of victimization.

Tiger's eye - This golden stone boosts power and motivation. It releases fear and anxiety and self-doubt, which improves your chance at career success. Helps you to make clear, conscious decisions.

Moonstone - Moonstone is known for bringing new beginnings. It encourages personal growth and develops inner strength. Moonstone can soothe stressful feelings when the way seems blocked. It promotes a positive attitude and brings inspiration, helping you to achieve good fortune and success.

Apatite - This highly energizing stone will fill you with passion for all creative pursuits, for life, and achievement. Your sense of self-expression will be clear and focussed. You will know what you want in life, and a job, and you will be energized and committed to achieving just that. Apatite will help you to feel inspired and ready to embrace the new.

Chrysocolla - When you are stuck in the dreaming phase, and struggling to get to the action phase, Chrysocolla is the right stone for you. Chrysocolla will fill you with willpower, energy, and confidence to take those dreams and make them real. It's the right stone to bring with you into a new job, helping to make it everything that you want.

Green Calcite - Green calcite raises your vibration to that of abundance so that you can bring your intentions to fruition. Green calcite improves communication, determination, and balance. This stone will give you the confidence to move forward into a positive new experience.

Kambaba Jasper - This dark, mystical, swirling stone gives you the strength to overcome your fears and anxieties. You will have a calm clarity and confidence about what you have to offer the world. You will be both thrilled and terrified as Kambaba Jasper guides you onto a whole new path.

Lepidolite - Through steady progress, Lepidolite will move you into your next adventure, from chaos to order. Lepidolite helps you to adjust your vibration to enter the new with ease.

Pyrite - Pyrite is also called fool's gold because it looks so similar to real gold. Pyrite helps to draw in real abundance. It is protective while showing you what needs to change for you to raise your vibration to the point where you are quickly attracting that which you desire.

Rhyolite - Do you find that you are stuck in the past, either wishing that you were still living that old life, or stuck in regrets of past decisions? Rhyolite is the stone to help you peacefully leave your past behind you. The stone will help to boost your self-esteem and helps you to release emotional attachment to the past. Rhyolite helps you to use the lessons of the past to build a joy-filled, positive future, helping you to now that everything will work out.

Agate - The magic of Agate is that it fills you with positivity and hope for the future. Agate is an excellent stone for assessing the pros and cons of any opportunities so that you can move forward with confidence.

Also, see Crystals for Getting that Promotion which can help you to draw success towards your job searching endeavors.

Numbers for finding a good job

Number one - This energy brings confidence. Number one aligns your frequency with creation and new beginnings. As the first whole number, this is the energy of new beginnings, confidence, and focussed intentions. When working with the power of one, be sure that you are clear about what it is you want. The one energy will direct your vibration based on your recurring thoughts. Be sure that your thoughts are focussed on what you do want.

Number Five - The five energy represents fresh starts, adventure, excitement, and freedom. It is the most dynamic of the single-digit numbers, and therefore always needing constant change.

Number Ten - Number ten marks the end of a cycle, and the opportunity for fresh starts and surprise wealth.

Number Fifty-Five - Number fifty-five helps you to release everything that no longer serves you. It helps you to release fear and doubt so that you can raise your vibration to the place that will welcome in the new.

Colors for finding a good job

Green - The color of growth and abundance, green brings prosperity, employment, renewal and wealth, ideal to wear when looking for a new job. Burn a green candle for new beginnings, employment opportunities, especially in the creative or natural fields, abundance, career growth, and inner peace.

Gold - This magical color brings inner strength and clarity. Gold brings success and good fortune. Wear golden jewelry to all job interviews. Gold also guides your intuition so stay alert for signs and positive feelings.

Orange is excellent for attracting new opportunities into your life. Orange is the color of creativity and self-expression, helping you to write your resume, or to best express what you have to offer in an interview. Orange also lightens the mood, which is helpful if you are feeling stressed about job seeking. Orange improves mental alertness and material gain.

Angels and Deities for finding a good job

Archangel Gabriel - As the messenger Angel, Archangel Gabriel can help you to best express yourself, and also to bring new opportunities to you if you ask.

Archangel Chamuel - Call on Archangel Chamuel to develop long-lasting relationships in your career, so that they are joyful and meaningful. With Archangel Chamuel, you may find that you receive an offer from a previous employer.

Lu-Hsing - This ascended master takes care of career progress, increases, employment, and a steady increase of wealth over time. Lu-Hsing is one of the three powerful Chine deities, collectively called the 'Fu Lu Shou San Hsing.' They bring joy, health, and long life. Call on Lu-Hsing to bring a new job, job interviews, and career growth.

Archangel Chamuel - Chamuel means 'he who seeks God.' He will help you to find the right job that aligns with your life purpose, and that is fulfilling for you. Call on Archangel Chamuel to bring an abundant salary with that job.

Archangel Michael - Archangel Michael's name means "he who is like God." He can help you to find work that is fulfilling and aligned to your purpose, especially if that action benefits the world. He builds your feelings of self-worth and courage so that you know how deserving you are of having work that is meaningful, joyful, and abundant.

Archangel Jehudiel vibrates at the frequency that gives you divine direction. He can help you to build your self-esteem and confidence. This vibration opens you up to work that you will enjoy. Jehudiel brings success in your career.

Archangel Gazardiel is also known as "the illuminated one." who can illuminate your way. Gazardiel can help you when you want to start a new career.

Switch Words for finding a good job

ACT - Increases motivation and releases stagnation and procrastination. This switchword raises your performance, triumph, and reaction time.

AMBER - This switchword releases all negative emotions and increases your positivity. AMBER heals emotional pain and stress so that you can bring in what you desire.

AMAZING - This switchword will bring in miracles that bring you joy and gratitude. It is used to create extreme miracles.

BRING - This Master Switchword helps to bring your goals to you much more quickly.

CIRCULATE - Keeps energy flowing and attracts new beginnings. CIRCULATE also markets your name so that the right jobs come to you more easily.

COUNT - brings in abundance and releases poverty. Inspires you to take the right steps towards success.

CREATE - Helps you to start something new, and attracts opportunities towards you.

DAWN - Brings faith that new beginnings are possible, lights your path and helps you to know that the good is coming.

FIND ADD COUNT TOGETHER - This SWP brings new opportunities and new income streams. FIND ADD COUNT TOGETHER helps to bring elements that will increase abundance, be that a new job, more clients, more sales.

FLOWER - With FLOWER, you can attract good fortune and wealth. It can open you up to receiving all that is good.

GANESHA - The elephant-headed god helps to attract new beginnings, wealth, remove obstacles, increase knowledge.

NOW - This master switchword can speed up the manifestation of what you desire. It increases momentum in your life, shifts procrastination, and inspires action in a calm, clear-headed manner. NOW releases old blocks and trauma that could be holding you back. Use NOW along with GOLDEN SUNRISE to bring in a new job.

GOLDEN SUNRISE EASE NOW - If you're stuck in the mode of complaining, feeling sorry for yourself, repeated negative thoughts, this is a powerful SWP to release this. This SWP will raise your vibration to the point where good things can flow to you. With this SWP, you will see more things to be grateful for and blocks will clear from your path.

NEXT - This helps you to move quickly to the next task. Keeps your focus on the action steps that will bring in the new. Completion of the old so that you can move forward smoothly.

SUDDENLY - Speeds up the pace and brings quick results. Can change a situation immediately. It brings unexpected success.

VICTORY - Fills you with the courage and confidence to achieve your desires, allowing good things to flow to you.

Booster Switch Words

DIVINE MAGIC BEGIN NOW - With this switch word phrase (SWP), we surrender to Divine powers. We ask them to begin their magic to fulfill our wishes and to manifest our desires with the Divine grace, love, and care. Use this SWP for any desire.

GOLDEN SUNRISE BRING MAGIC - This SWP calls on GOLDEN SUNRISE a very powerful SWP to begin blessing us right now with divine flow. Think about what you want to achieve while using this SWP, and it can flow to you more quickly.

ADD - This master switchword brings more power and strength to whatever you focus on, and helps to promote anything.

SPEED - Quickens the manifestation of abundance and success

CHEERS - increases happiness, joy, good luck, and success. Especially useful for the positive outcome of any event.

AIM - Helps to keep you focused on the goal for a successful outcome.

BRING, TOGETHER - Improves your ability to manifest that which you want

DIVINE - This switchword brings in the miraculous

Creating a Sigil to find a good job

To begin creating your sigil, write out a positive statement
that reflects your specific desire. It should be in the present
tense, so starting with I AM / I HAVE helps. It should only
use positive words. Remember, you can use the sigil that I
have created below, but it would be far more powerful to
create your own sigil. By weaving your focused intention into
you sigil, you send a direct message of your intent to your
subconscious.

An example would be -

I HAVE A WONDERFUL NEW JOB WITH WONDERFUL
PAY

Remove all vowels

HVWNDRFLNWJBWTHWNDRFLPY

Remove any duplicated letters

HVWNDRFLJBTPY

Draw a sigil using the shapes of the remaining letters. Below
is an example of a sigil using the above phrase. You can use
this sigil, either as it is, or as inspiration. Remembering that it
is so much more powerful for you to create your own sigil.

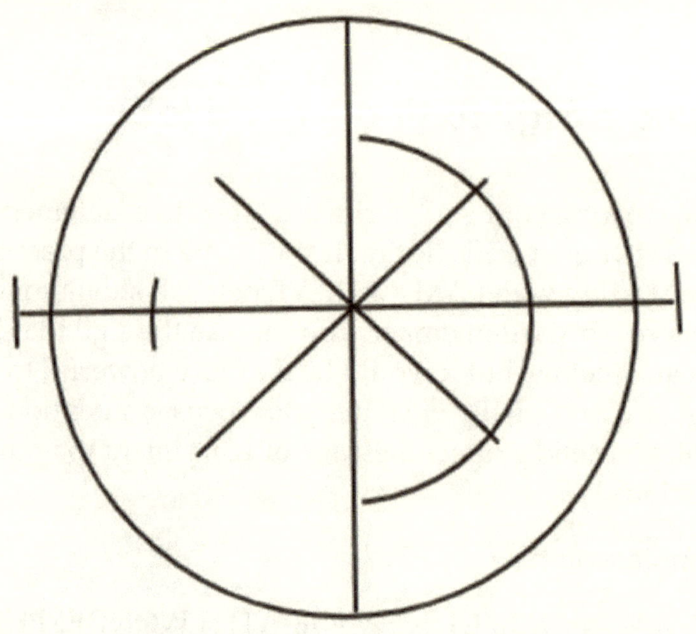

Creating your Energy Circle to attract a good job

Here is an example of an Energy Circle created to attract a good job. I would add a drop of camphor to my energy circle to concentrate the energies.

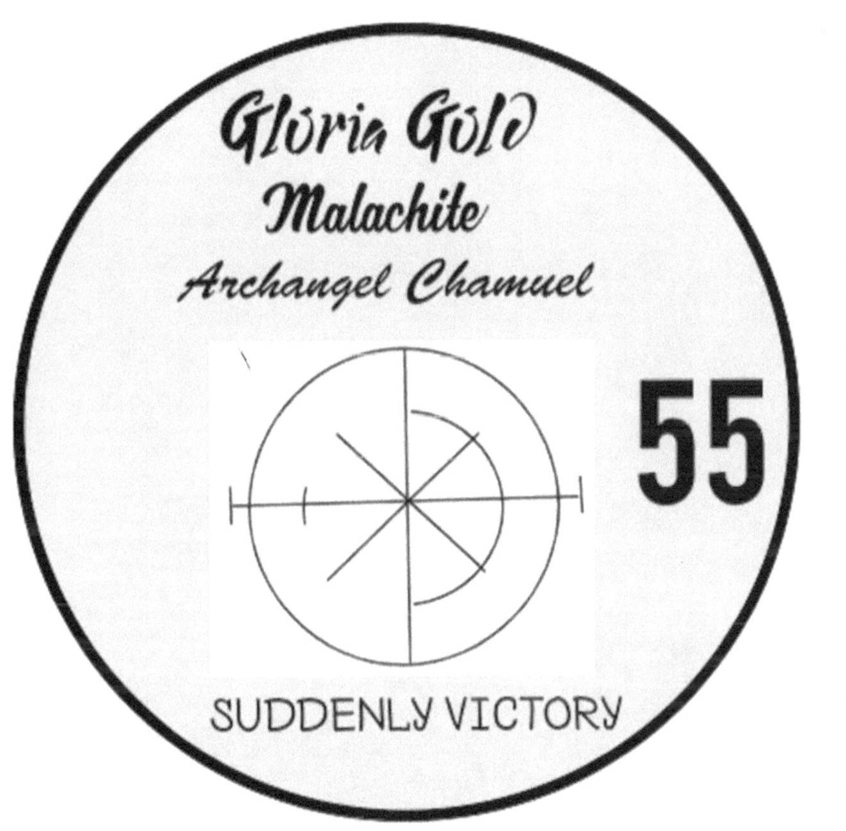

Vibrational Energy to bring more Joy to your Job

Like most people, you probably spend most of your daylight hours at your workplace. Vibrational energy can help you to make these hours meaningful and joyful by lifting your spirits, relieving stress and helping you to see the best in situations. Vibrational energy can help you to be recognised for your efforts and more. If it's office politics that's messing with your mojo, I cover that in it's own section later in the book.

Clarifying your request

What kind of work environment brings out the best in you?

What state of mind do you want to be in at work?

What emotional state do you want to have at work?

How do you want to contribute at work?

How do you want to engage with your colleagues?

What makes you feel valued and appreciated?

What else will make you enjoy your workplace more?

If any of these answers make you feel uncomfortable, work through that, or adjust the question and your response, until you have an unmistakable, joyful feeling when you think about receiving this promotion.

Write your clear desire down, and you can add, 'this or better now comes to me.'

Use this statement and joyful feeling when selecting and working with the energy tools that follow.

Essential Oils for bringing more joy to your job

Peony - This good luck oil attracts new positions, new customers, and good luck.

Lotus - This high vibration oil, used in ancient Egypt, is still used today for blessings, anointing, healing, and meditation. Wearing lotus oil brings happiness and good fortune.

Orange - This sweet, sharp scented oil made from orange rinds brings joy and ease to life. Place a few drops of orange oil into a diffuser to uplift your workspace.

Frankincense - This oil brings a centered calmness and a deeper connection to your spirit — ideal for easing stressful work environments.

Pine - This fresh scent helps you to see the best in those around you. Pine promotes a feeling of abundance and helps you to recognize and appreciate all the good in your life.

Cinnamon - This spicy scent invokes courage and happiness. It will help you to explore work that brings you joy, which may sometimes mean a change in career.

Ylang Ylang - This exotic floral scent helps to release anger and frustration. It can open you to forgiveness, which often releases the blocks to appreciation.

Lemon - This citrus scent helps to relieve stress, anger, and exhaustion. It brings calm and helps you to move forward with positivity.

Lavender - This relaxing oil relieves nervous tension and lifts depression, helping you to see the good around you. Lavender is excellent at relieving stress-related headaches and migraines.

Jasmine - This calming oil acts as an antidepressant. It can revive a low spirit helping you to feel optimistic, confident, and energized.

Crystals and Gemstones for bringing more joy to your job

Citrine - Often called the "Success Stone" or the "Merchant's Stone"; Citrine brings joy and positivity. Citrine works on your solar plexus chakra to improve your sense of self-worth and increase your power. Citrine clears negative energies in the environment. Citrine can help to bring you balance by absorbing and removing the vibration of depression and bad moods.

Amethyst - This calming stone helps you to relax and release pent up stress. This purple vibration works on your third eye chakra, helping you to see past the negative emotions to better resolve your challenges. This nurturing, nourishing stone helps you to unwind after too many stresses. Amethyst helps clear and energize your third eye and your crown chakra. It helps to calm you to see past the emotion towards the right solution to your challenges.

Fluorite - This crystal absorbs all negative energy in your vibration and the environment around you. Your energy will be cleared and filled with joy and peace. Fluorite absorbs anxiety and brings tranquility.

Garnet stimulates your life force and energizes you to embrace all that life has to offer. This stone clears all blocks that are holding you back from living your best life. With a boost from garnet, everything is possible.

Ocean Jasper washes away stress and leaves you filled with positivity. In challenging times, Ocean Jasper gives you the insight to achieve a peaceful outcome with sensitivity and ease.

Red Jasper - This grounding stone brings a sense of security and love. It helps you to feel cared for and nurtured in stressful times. Red Jasper soothes your mind so that you have the breathing space to shift your thoughts and energies to a more positive vibration.

Smoky Quartz - This crystal gets you out of a funk and into the light. Smoky Quartz helps you to shift out of depression, resentment, anger and jealousy so that you feel lighter and more able to move forward.

Numbers for bringing more joy to your job

Number Fifty brings positivity and joy.

Number Three - This vibration improves teamwork. It is a social energy that opens people up to being more generous and playful with each other. The three helps to shift office energy to the light.

Colors for bringing more joy to your job

Yellow is the joyful color of sunshine. The right bright yellow impacts the solar plexus chakra, which is all about self-identity and immediately lifts the spirits by making you feel confident and positive about yourself.

Blue brings a calming effect and encourages ease of speaking and self-expression. The primary shade of blue is great for lifting mood in a calming and secure way.

Green is made up of yellow and blue, and so vibrates with aspects of each of these colors. Green resonates with the heart chakra and can improve feelings of love and open-heartedness. It is also the color that vibrates with abundance and promotes feelings of financial ease which can bring joy to the workplace.

Angels and Deities for bringing more joy to your job

Archangel Gabriel - Helps you to find your passion, and supports you in following your dreams.

Archangel Haniel - As the Archangel of energy and vitality, call on Archangel Haniel to raise all lower vibration energies and bring you back to a place of love.

Archangel Jophiel - Helps you to move your focus from the things that are not working onto everything good and positive in your work experience. The more you can focus your thoughts and feelings on what is right, the more you will draw similar energies into your life.

Switch Words for bringing more joy to your job

BUFFER - Protects you from harmful people and stressful situations. BUFFER brings stability in finance and career.

BUZZ - Brings excitement, and high energy to complete tasks efficiently.

CHAMOMILE - Brings good luck and a positive, winning attitude. It clears all negativity and curses from your environment.

CHEERS - Increases good luck and joy. It brings positivity and encouragement.

DELIVER - Helps to get tasks completed well and on time. This switchword brings in hope and optimism.

DYNAMIC - Increases energy, confidence, and mental vibrancy. Charges and refreshes.

ELM - This switchword comes from the Bach flower remedy, elm. Use ELM to increase your self-confidence, and to feel that you can take responsibility. Releases feelings of being overwhelmed and anxious. It brings focus and clarity.

FLASH - Brings some light into the darkness with a burst. Can boost career growth and give you an energetic charge — short term super booster.

GIGGLE STRETCH BLUFF - This SWP releases depression and stress. It makes space for joy and happiness to flow.

GOLDEN SUNRISE DONE - This SWP helps to successfully and efficiently complete a project and to solve challenges.

HAVEN - Creates a safe and peaceful environment. Brings in divine help and opens up new opportunities.

NEXT - Helps to complete tasks that need concentration and focused attention. NEXT brings in new opportunities.

ON - Energises and expands your thinking and attitude towards work. Inspires new thinking and new solutions. Can help to keep a project on track and moving forward.

OPEN - Clears the old so that new opportunities can come to you. Helps to release resistance and fear. OPEN brings a feeling of lightness, joy, and possibility. Helps to embrace change.

PASSION - Increases determination and commitment to completing a task. Increases focus. It brings joy and enthusiasm to tasks.

PERFECT - Improves all aspects of your life. PERFECT brings job satisfaction. It helps you to deliver high-quality work within deadlines to exceed the expectations of your superiors at work.

PLAY - Makes work easy and fun. PLAY brings enthusiasm and an open-minded attitude.

PRAISE - Increases your sense of self-worth and releases both internal and external criticism. It brings in praise, recognition, and compliments.

PRECIOUS - Increases your feelings of self-worth. It brings in praise and recognition. PRECIOUS helps you to feel respected and valued at work, and increases the value that you bring to your company.

QUENCH - Brings completion to tasks so that you can enjoy relief and a break from work.

RELISH - Fully enjoy every experience. It brings delight and much happiness.

RHYTHM - Brings flow. Allows for work to become more manageable and for you to become more efficient. RHYTHM increases peace and happiness to make you feel fulfilled.

STAR - Shows you the way to achieve success with wisdom. Improves your work performance and attracts appreciation for your high-quality work.

WALNUT LETTING GO DONE - This SWP helps you to shift from a negative experience into a positive future. Clears old energy so that you can confidently make decisions without past fears holding you back. This SWP releases confusion and clears negative influence from others.

WAVE - Keeps you calm, focused, and energized. Allows you to be in flow. Very energizing makes you an unstoppable force of achievement and positivity.

WILD OAT - This switchword comes from the Bach flower remedy. Releases frustration and confusion. It brings clarity about the best way forward. Brings commitment to your decisions so that you can achieve your goals.

WILLOW - Another Bach flower remedy switchword. It clears your vibration from feeling victimized, from blaming, and from comparing yourself to others. WILLOW restores your energy to vitality. Releases feelings of bitterness, and brings in light for a more balanced life.

Creating a Sigil to bring more joy to your job

To begin creating your sigil, write out a positive statement that reflects your specific desire. It should be in the present tense, so starting with I AM helps. It should only use positive words. Remember, you can use the sigil that I have created below. It would be more potent for you to create your sigil. Your focused intention is woven into the sigil, sending a direct message of your intent to your subconscious.

An example would be -

I AM SO SUPPORTED, VALUED AND APPRECIATED IN MY JOB

Remove all vowels

MSSPPRTDVLDNDPPRCTDNMYJB

Remove any duplicated letters

MSPRTDVLNCYJB

Draw a sigil using the shapes of the remaining letters. Below is an example of a sigil using the above phrase. You can use this sigil, either as it is, or as inspiration. Remembering that it is so much more powerful for you to create your own sigil.

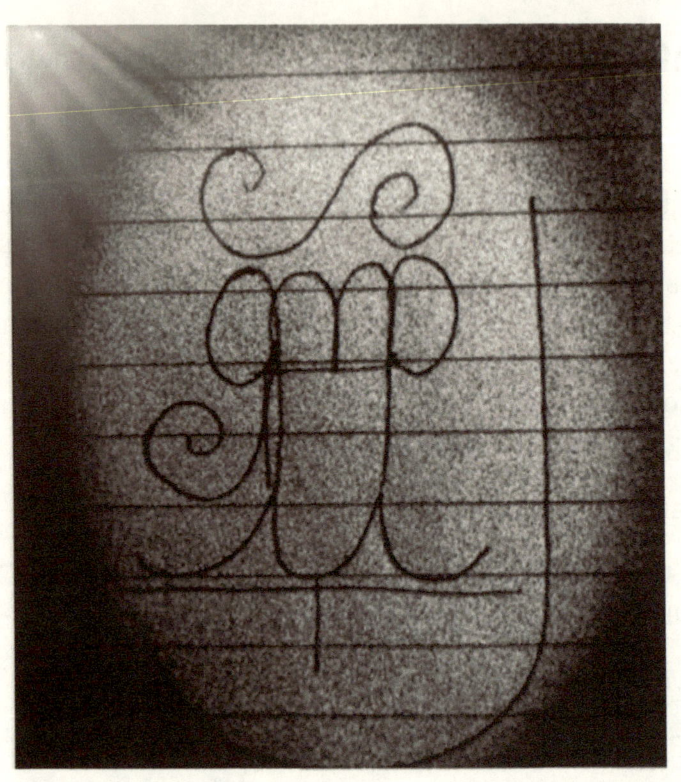

Creating your Energy Circle to bring more joy to your job

Here is an example of an Energy Circle created to bring more joy to your job. A drop or two of cinnamon will also help to boost this energy circle.

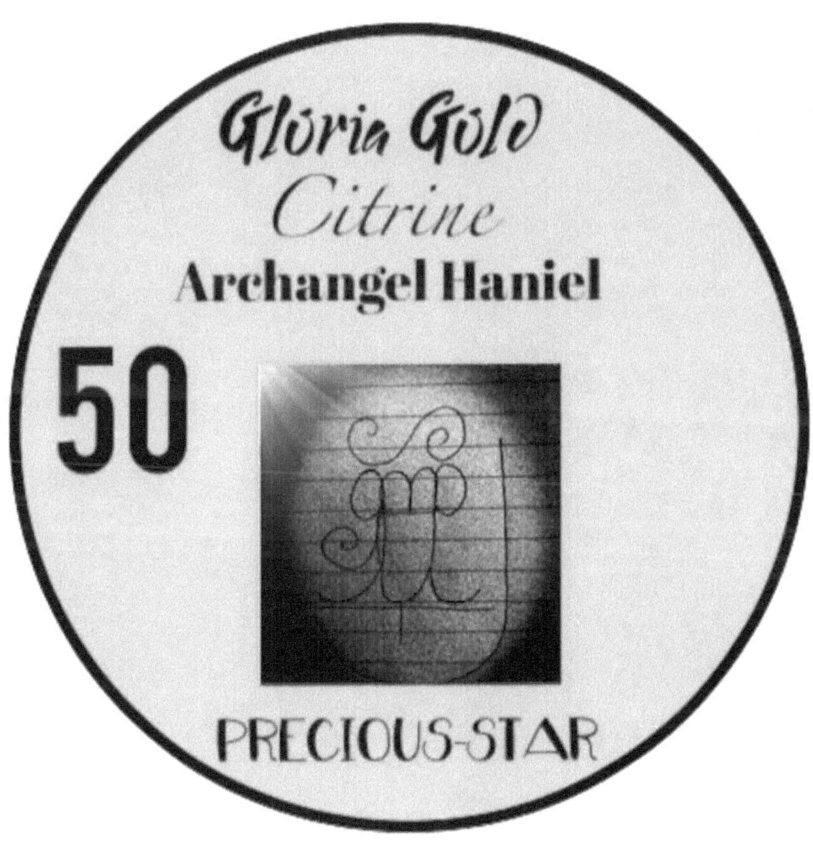

Vibrational Energy to Boost Creativity

You don't have to be an artist or a writer to bring creativity to your role. You can tap into creativity when you need to solve a problem, address a workplace challenge, come up with a new product or service offering, write a report, and so much more.

Clarifying your request

Which areas of your role require a creative approach?

Where do you feel stuck in your role, that you feel some creativity could help you get into flow?

What other aspects of creativity would help you to shine at work?

If any of these answers make you feel uncomfortable, work through that, or adjust the question and your response, until you have an unmistakable, joyful feeling when you think about receiving this promotion.

Write your clear desire down, and you can add, 'this or better now comes to me.'

Use this statement and joyful feeling when selecting and working with the energy tools that follow.

Essential Oils for boosting creativity

Essential oils are especially powerful at boosting creativity, as they help to reduce stress and anxiety, and raise your levels of serotonin and dopamine, the feel-good chemicals. Leonardo Da Vinci was said to use the scents of plants to stimulate creativity, with his favorite being the heady citrus scent of Neroli.

Vervain (Verbena) - This oil helps to overcome creative blocks, and to keep you calm and inspired when a deadline is looming.

Frankincense - This earthy, slightly sweet scented oil de-stresses you, without creating sleepiness. This oil will also lower anxiety and improve mood.

Neroli - This floral-citrus oil improves mood and reduces stress. It adds a real zing of positivity which can help to create a sense of safety to express and explore creative ideas without fear of criticism or judgment.

Jasmine - This heady floral fragrance is calming and emotionally balancing. It increases confidence and creativity.

Ylang Ylang - This sweet, floral fragrance is a sensual and mentally exhilarating oil. It inspires creativity and can help you shift from dullness to enthusiasm.

Crystals and Gemstones for boosting creativity

Sunstone - This red speckled stone feeds your sacral and solar plexus energy centers, bringing self-confidence, vitality, and leadership energy. Like sunshine, the Sun Stone brings hope and joy and life.

Sodalite - When you're feeling stuck in a non-creative rut, Sodalite will awaken your creative energies and bring out your full creative talent.

Amazonite - Use Amazonite when the pain from the past, even a recent negative experience, causes your vibration to drop, blocking joy and confidence. Amazonite floods your heart and throat chakras with joy and love. Amazonite helps you to release hurt and darkness so that you can allow joy back in. Some artists and writers feel that creativity can come from a dark emotional space, but workplace creativity tends to come from a place of energy and lightness, which is the energy of Amazonite.

Apatite- This highly energizing stone will fill you with passion for all creative pursuits, for life, and achievement. Your sense of self-expression will be clear and focussed.

Chrysocolla - When you are stuck in the dreaming phase, and struggling to get to the action phase, Chrysocolla is the right stone for you. Chrysocolla will fill you with willpower, energy, and confidence to express your creativity.

Carnelian - This stone sends a powerful burst of energy to your sacral chakra, helping you to feel creative and confident. With Carnelian, you will be able to break through creative blocks. The sure power that Carnelian brings will help you to express your creativity within the workplace.

Numbers for boosting creativity

Zero (Nought) - Zero is the emptiness and the whole; it is the non-number which creates. Creative doodling often involves versions of the zero and is a beneficial number at the start of a creative process when the big idea is needed.

One - Because of the confidence and leadership qualities of number one, it can help creativity by making you more certain of yourself, and feeling confident enough to share your ideas. The caution would be that it can make you feel that your idea is the only right one, and you may be resistant to other people's creative contribution.

Three is an organized number, as well as offering intelligence and humorous spark. Useful for coming up with marketing messages and for challenges that need quick, smart solutions.

Nine - This humanitarian number removes ego and replaces it with childlike wonder, and love for all. Nine is a useful frequency to tap into for a creative solution to a social challenge, extending thinking beyond self and into a broader, universal mindset.

Colors for boosting creativity

Orange - This energizing vibration is the color of creativity and self-expression. Orange will help you to get through a creative block, allowing ideas to flow freely again.

Yellow - The bright color of sunshine will give your creativity a boost. Yellow relieves stuffy, slow thinking, and brings energy and inspiration.

Angels and Deities for boosting creativity

Shakti - The divine feminine energy is the force of creativity. Shakti energy inspires life and vibrates in all things.

The Goddess Danu / Anu - This Irish goddess is the mother of creativity, abundance, love, and wisdom. She is the patron saint of creativity. As the goddess of waters, she brings the ebb and flow of inspiration.

The Creative Forest Goddess Sadv - This forest goddess brings sun-dappled forest creativity. Gentle inspiration on the soft breeze - this is the energy that you can access when connecting with Sadv.

Saraswati - She is the Hindu goddess of flowing waters, the arts, music, nature, and wisdom. She brings free flowing inspiration and allows your creativity and intellect to merge and support each other.

Ix Chel (Ixchel) - This Mayan deity of creativity will unlock your creativity, especially at the beginning of a new project. Ixchel helps you to release control of outcomes so that your creative juices flow more freely and spontaneously.

Switchwords for boosting creativity

ON - For increased creativity

ARCHANGEL GABRIEL - Use this Archangel's name as a switchword to feel motivated, creative, and inspired. She brings strength to artists.

CHISEL - Benefits all creatives in the arts. Helps to bring the ordinary into the extraordinary.

ORANGE - This color switchword brings creative thinking, and frees the body and mind from restrictions, allowing enthusiasm and expression. ORANGE also brings abundance and success and celebration. Note - Be careful not to overuse the switchword ORANGE as this may leave you feeling irritable, frustrated, and hungry!

UNPLUG - Shifts you beyond restrictive or limited thinking so that new solutions and big ideas can flow. Also helps you to separate from the world for a while. Can remove obstacles.

VUM - The seed mantra of the sacral chakra. Increases creativity, fun, and a sense of self-worth. Clears and charges the sacral chakra.

WHIMSICAL - Makes odd ideas pop up suddenly. It brings innovative, never been done before solutions forward. Used on a person, this creates the vibration of joy and being unusual and fantastical.

WIND - Powerful creative energy. Brings a blast of energy to make a substantial impact and do exceptionally well. The strength of expansiveness and clarity brings out the extraordinary.

Creating a Sigil to boost creativity

To begin creating your sigil, write out a positive statement that reflects your specific desire. It should be in the present tense, so starting with I AM helps. It should only use positive words. Remember, you can use the sigil that I have created below. It would be more potent for you to create your sigil, sending a direct message of your intent to your subconscious.

An example would be -

I AM A POWERFUL CREATIVE BEING

Remove all vowels

MPWRFLCRTVBNG

Remove any duplicated letters

MPWRFLCTVBNG

Draw a sigil using the shapes of the remaining letters. Below is an example of a sigil using the above phrase. You can use this sigil, either as it is, or as inspiration. Remembering that it is so much more powerful for you to create your own sigil.

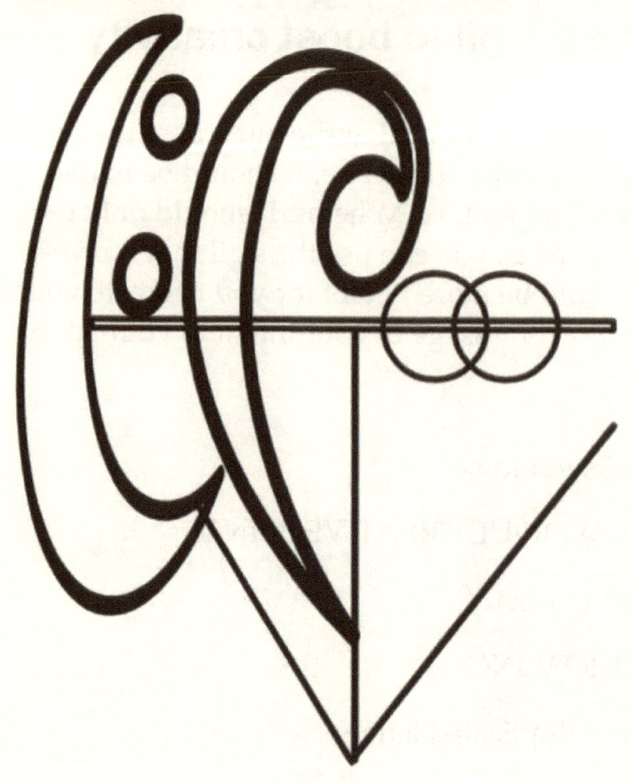

Creating your Energy Circle to boost creativity

Here is an example of an Energy Circle created to boost your creativity.

I would also add a few drops of ylang ylang and a drop of verbena.

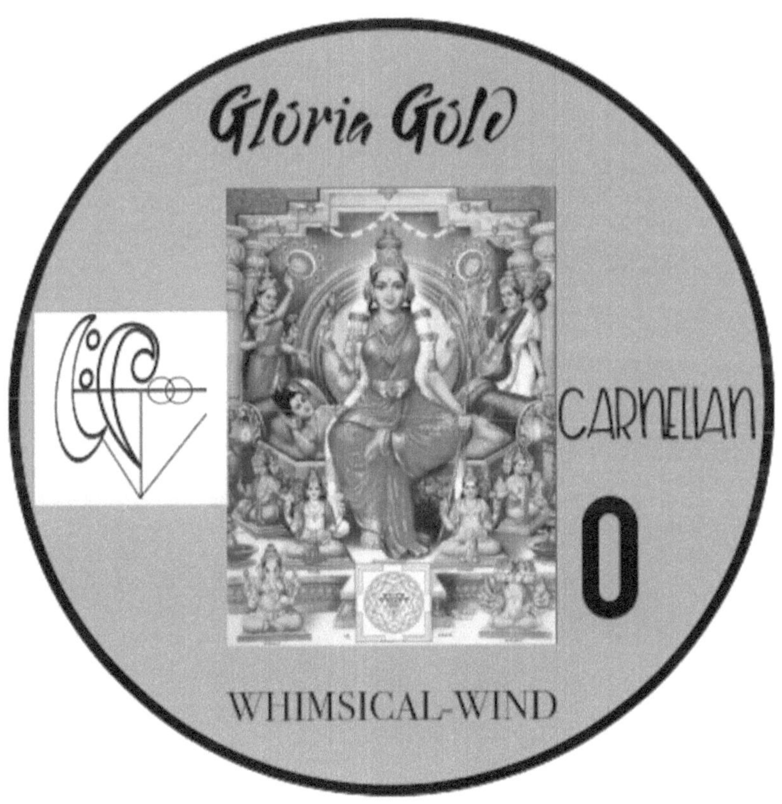

Vibrational Energy to get a Good Pay Increase

Vibrational energy can help you to get a pay increase by raising your vibration to one of abundance, increasing your luck, improving your ability to manifest, increasing your self worth and releasing you from past experiences that tell you otherwise.

Clarifying your request

Exactly how much would you like to earn?

What percent increase is this from your current income?

Would you like this money to come from the same source, i.e. your current job?

Would you like this income to come from a different source? If so, which source?

How will you use this additional income?

Is there anything else that would help you to clarify your desire?

If any of these answers make you feel uncomfortable, work through that, or adjust the question and your response, until you have an unmistakable, joyful feeling when you think about receiving this promotion.

Write your clear desire down, and you can add, 'this or better now comes to me.'

Use this statement and joyful feeling when selecting and working with the energy tools that follow.

Essential Oils to get a good pay increase

Bayberry - This oil brings 'luck into your home, and gold into your pocket.' Rub a few drops onto a green candle, starting at the center and rubbing outwards to each end. Light the candle stating your desired income, along with an expected timeline. Let the candle burn right down.

Bergamot - This citrus scented oil brings abundance. Rub a few drops onto the palms of your hands to draw in prosperity.

Hyssop - This woody-camphorus scented oil draws in money. Hyssop can help you to release all negative beliefs that you have around lack so that you are more easily able to match an abundance vibration.

Mint - Add a few drops of mint to your wallet to increase your cash flow. Mint oil is excellent for business success and prosperity spells.

Caraway - This sweet and spicy aromatic oil brings good luck and prosperity.

Cedarwood oil is excellent for purification, protection and wealth. Keep a piece of Cedarwood in your purse to attract money.

Nutmeg - This spicy oil is excellent for luck and attracts money. Use in prosperity spells.

The following oils and herbs all assist in drawing money to you - Allspice, Almond, Basil, Bergamot Mint, Calamus, Chamomile, Cedarwood, Cinnamon, Cinquefoil, Clove, Clover, Dill, Elder, Galangal, Ginger, Heliotrope, Honeysuckle, Hyssop, Jasmine, Myrtle, Nutmeg, Oakmoss, Orange, Patchouli, Peppermint, Periwinkle, Pine, Sage, Sassafras, Tonka, Vanilla, Vervain, Vetivert, Wood Aloe, Woodruff.

Also see 'Getting a Promotion' and 'Getting a job' for more abundance drawing oils.

Crystals and Gemstones to get a good pay increase

Mookaite - This amber-hued stone brings material success while keeping you grounded.

Pyrite - This protective stone deflects negativity away from you. It brings luck and helps to attract abundance. Pyrite has intense manifestation energy, so be clear about your desires when programming Pyrite.

Citrine - This "Success Stone" brings good fortune and good luck in the most unexpected ways. Citrine brings success and abundance, especially in business. Citrine is a self-clearing stone and absorbs then clears all negativity both within and around you.

Malachite - This vibrant green stone can be used to transform beliefs of lack into abundance, helping you to create a significant increase in wealth.

Gold Stone - This manufactured stone is speckled with gold flecks and brings good luck and good fortunes.

Jade - This beautiful gem brings good luck. Jade opens you up to receive prosperity and abundance. Tapping into ancient wisdom, Jade can help you see your challenges from a much broader perspective. Jade brings a sense of peace which allows you to see through stress and tension to have a clear vision of who you can be.

Also see 'Getting a Promotion' and 'Getting a job' for more abundance drawing stones.

Numbers to get a good pay increase

Number Eight. The eight brings in wealth and financial sensibility. If you have been overspending or struggling to manage your budget, call on the power of eight, and soon enough, your income will be higher than your expenditure. Eight rewards you for the work and effort that you put in.

Colors to get a good pay increase

Green. The color of nature, the heart chakra, and abundance. In the way that an acorn grows into a great tree, green brings steady financial growth. Green is also the color of good luck, and you can experience some surprise blessings when working with green.

Gold brings a naturally abundant energy, use gold in your office as a picture frame or other ornament, and keep something gold in your wallet for financial abundance.

Angels and Deities to get a good pay increase

Gazardiel - This Archangel brings in salary increases and new work opportunities. Call on Gazardiel if you need to receive a pay increase.

Lakshmi - Call on the Hindu Goddess of beauty, abundance, and good fortune to help you draw in prosperity and wealth. Lakshmi can increase your income and help you to grow prosperous. There are beautiful mantras that you can chant to honor this Deity.

Abundantia - This beautiful Roman goddess brings success and prosperity. She also protects your savings and investments. She loves to help if you call on her, and loves the gratitude that someone feels after receiving her help. She alleviates your low vibration thoughts of scarcity and helps you to prosper.

Switchwords to get a good pay increase

ADD - Increases anything

BRING, TOGETHER - Manifestation

COUNT - This strong switchword attracts money and releases poverty.

87 RAISE PROFITS - This SWP helps to increase sales and your income.

ADD - This Master Switchword increases and adds power to any request, increasing it in size.

ADD COUNT MAGIC NOW - Use this SWP to increase your salary quickly.

ADD COUNT TOGETHER - This SWP improves your financial condition by helping you to align your thoughts positively around money.

BONUS - Use BONUS if you feel that you need more reward for your hard work. BONUS can also bring unexpected money and abundance.

CLAP - This switchword ensures that you are appreciated for the work that you do, thereby helping you to secure that increase.

FLOWER - This switchword helps to make you prosperous and opens you up to receiving good fortune.

GOLDEN SUNRISE ADD COUNT NOW - This SWP helps to increase wealth opportunity, increase earning, abundance, and more cash flow.

REACH FIND DIVINE COUNT - This SWP calls on divine help to attract the salary that you desire.

Creating a Sigil to get a good pay increase

To begin creating your sigil, write out a positive statement that reflects your specific desire. It should be in the present tense, so starting with I AM helps. It should only use positive words. Remember, you can use the sigil that I have created below, but it would be far more powerful to create your sigil. Your sigil weaves your focused intention into the sigil, making the sigil send a direct message of your intent to your subconscious.

An example would be -

I AM VERY WELL REWARDED FOR MY WORK

Remove all vowels

MVRYWLLRWRDDFRMYWRK

Remove any duplicated letters

MVRYWLDFK

Draw a sigil using the shapes of the remaining letters. Below is an example of a sigil using the above phrase. You can use this sigil, either as it is, or as inspiration. Remembering that it is so much more powerful for you to create your own sigil.

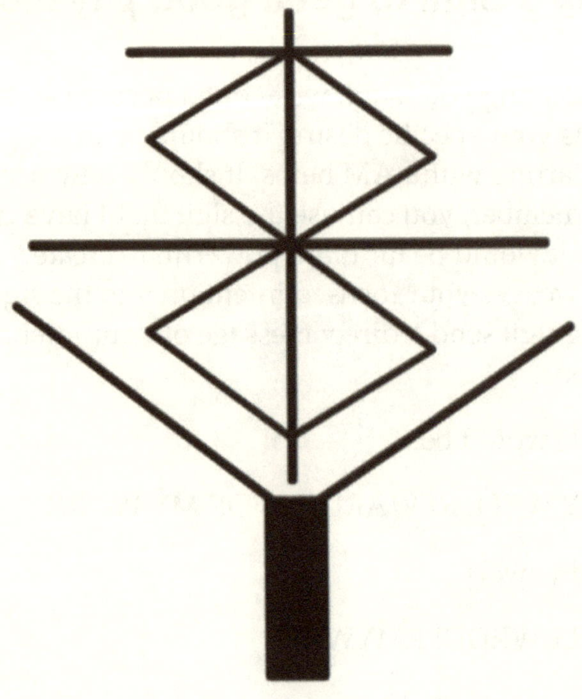

Creating your Energy Circle to get a good pay increase

Here is an example of an Energy Circle created to attract a pay increase.

I would also add a drop of nutmeg and a drop of caraway into my energy circle.

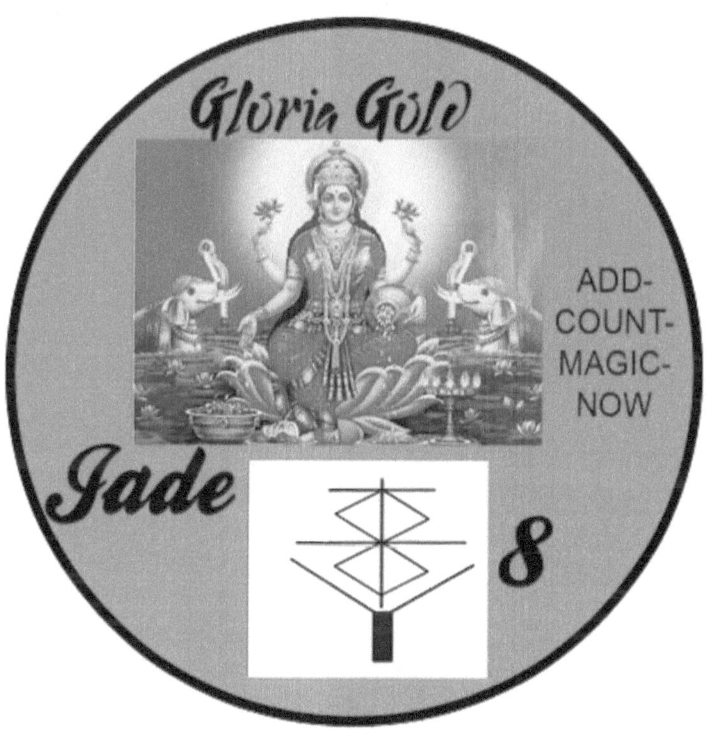

Vibrational Energy to clear Office Politics

Office politics can be really stressful and can lower your vibration, thereby impacting many other aspects of your wellbeing. You can use vibrational energy very effectively to protect yourself from office politics, and to remove the stressful experience from your environment entirely.
You can use these tools to clear office politics between yourself and colleagues, or to clear the air between yourself and your boss.

Clarifying your request

What kind of office environment do you want to work in?

In the perfect environment, how will your colleagues treat you?

How will they speak to you?

What will they include you in?

What experiences will you have with them?

How would you like to feel waking up on a workday morning?

How would you like to feel on your way home from the office?

Is there anything else that will help to clarify your desire?

If any of these answers make you feel uncomfortable, work through that, or adjust the question and your response, until you have an unmistakable, joyful feeling when you think about receiving this promotion.

Write your clear desire down, and you can add, 'this or better now comes to me.'

Use this statement and joyful feeling when selecting and working with the energy tools that follow.

Essential Oils to clear office politics

Clove - Clove oil is perfect for stopping gossip; it purifies and raises vibrations.

Birch - Use this sweet, wintergreen fragrance oil to establish a positive connection with others; it brings peace and harmony.

Cumin Seed - Also known as Kulanji Oil or Black Seed Oil, this oil is a miracle worker on many levels. One vibrational aspect is that it brings peace and harmony into your environment. Place a few drops over each doorway of your office space so that all who enter may come in peace.

Basil - Wear Basil oil when you want to avoid a clash with someone. Basil oil brings empathy and harmony and helps to keep the peace. Basil oil has an overpowering scent, so use sparingly, blended with other lighter scents.

Narcissus - This oil has the smell of a forest, or many green leaves. It is also called the "Stupidfyer" as it soothes the nerves and relaxes your mind. Narcissus brings harmony. This oil is quite heady, so use sparingly.

Rue - Seen as a magical oil by many cultures; it can clear curses and release all negativity. This oil is powerful, smelly and quite toxic. It should not be used as an essential oil, but you can use it's name in your Energy Circle if you feel that negativity directed towards you is intentional (feels like you've been cursed).

Angelica - This woody-peppery scented oil brings peace and is wonderful for attracting friends and prosperity. Angelica is phototoxic, meaning that it causes a reaction when exposed to sunlight, giving you 'sunburn' and skin irritation, so don't use if you're planning to spend time in the sun.

Crystals and Gemstones to clear office politics

Ruby - Brings courage and strength and can help to increase your success in disputes and arguments.

Rose quartz - This gentle pink stone is all about love. Rose quartz can restore trust in all relationships. This stone brings harmony and deepens relationships.

Jasper is the "supreme nurturer" - it protects you from negative energies and gives you the courage to face challenging issues.

Citrine - Amongst its many uses, Citrine helps to clear the air of negative energies and restores balance and harmony. Citrine brings joy and positivity into your world and helps to relieve depression, anger, and self-doubt.

Black Onyx - This powerful black stone clears office rivalry. It protects you from negative energy directed at you and puts an end to any office gossip. If the gossip has nothing to do with you, Black Onyx will help you to stay focused on your work. Black Onyx ensures that you are not bothered by other people's drama.

Amazonite - By pouring loving energy into your heart and throat chakras, Amazonite will help you to clear old hurts and toxic negativity that has built up over time. Amazonite helps you to attract a peaceful, loving, supportive workplace and environment.

Black Tourmaline - This stone is a powerful protector and eliminator of negative energy. Black Tourmaline places a protective barrier between you and others, keeping you safe from negative energies. Place Black Tourmaline in each corner of your office space to form a protective shield that dispels low vibrations.

Bronzite - This dark golden stone returns all negative energy to the sender. It asks like a bronze shield keeping you protected. Bronzite also clears all chakras, ensuring that you are not a magnet for lower vibration energy.

Chrysoprase - This stone helps to resolve conflicts by opening the heart to see a broader perspective. Chrysoprase shifts petty judgments through love and kindness.

Peridot - This vibrant green stone brings light and helps you to release the energies of jealousy, spite, and stress. Once these energies are cleared, Peridot brings in confidence and a strong sense of purpose. You will be left feeling lighter and joyful, release from the grip of negativity.

Selenite - This translucent stone clears your environment brightening the space and everyone in it. Selenite cleanses and purifies, releasing all lower vibration energies.

Numbers to clear office politics

Number two brings harmony and union; it allows us to see both perspectives and to understand that there is more than one side to any story. Two is the number of Eve, the first woman, and brings the energy of wisdom and good judgment.

Number Twenty-Three - This number brings the energy of harmony, communication, and joy. It helps you to be diplomatic, boosts teamwork, and brings companionship.

Number Six - The six energy aims to bring peace and equilibrium between people. Six holds the vibration of peacemaker and negotiator.

Colors to clear office politics

Black clears negative energy from your space and brings transformation and enlightenment.

Grey helps you to reach a compromise.

Red brings bravery and strength when you do need to face conflict.

Sunshine yellow helps to persuade others of your point of view. It also brings protective energy. Yellow brings light and joy and raises the happiness levels in your environment.

Blue brings patience and understanding. Being the color of the throat chakra, it helps you to communicate clearly and authentically. It helps you to be open and honest and to open the lines of communication.

Angels and Deities to clear office politics

Archangel Gabriel - Call on Archangel Gabriel for strength and protection. Gabriel protects you from negativity and helps you to face difficult situations. Archangel Gabriel improves communication, especially in highly charged situations.

Archangel Orion - Call on Archangel Orion to clear the energy, and to release dark negative energy in the office. This Archangel raises your vibration so that you can see and appreciate all the good and beauty in your world.

Archangel Zadkiel - This Archangel of forgiveness radiates joy, love, forgiveness, freedom, and mercy. Using the violet flame of transmutation, Archangel Zadkiel will transmute all lower energies into light. Zadkiel will help you to release dark memories and emotions so that it is easier for you to find forgiveness and be open to joy again.

Archangel Raguel - Call on Raguel if you need help to create harmony and resolve conflicts.

Gavreel Angel of Peace - Gavreel helps you to find a way to make peace with your enemies.

Valoel Angel of Peace - Fills us with serenity and helps us to resolve conflicts with others.

Nemesis - This Greek goddess of retribution will help you to handle office politics and troublemakers. She will also help you to see where you are self-sabotaging.

Switchwords to clear office politics

CANCEL - Releases negativity.

SHINE - Raises your vibration and clears a negative atmosphere.

ABALONE - Changes negative energy into positive. Helps to control emotions and bring harmony.

ALIGN - Brings harmony by helping everyone to come into alignment and agreement.

ARCHANGEL RAGUEL - This Archangel switchword promotes justice and harmony. Raguel clears negativity and conflict and draws compatible people into your life.

CHANGE - This switchword can quickly change the energy to end arguments and remove negativity.

CHICORY - This Bach flower remedy raises the vibration of those who create drama to get attention. CHICORY also releases people from a false sense of victimization. CHICORY creates a loving, caring, sharing environment.

CONCEDE - This peacemaking switchword helps you to admit the truth. It can stop an argument and improve relationships. CONCEDE releases our attachment to being right and can help us to see the good around us.

EASE - This switchword creates comfort and helps to calm things down. EASE will release rigidity and free you from stressful people and situations.

GOLDEN SUNRISE HOLLY - This SWP helps to release anger and jealousy. It increases forgiveness and opens the heart to be more loving.

GOLDEN SUNRISE TOGETHER DIVINE - A master SWP that resolves all sorts of relationship challenges. It helps to get people talking to each other again and improves understanding.

HEATHER - This Bach flower remedy helps to manage over talkative and attention seekers.

HOLLY - This Bach flower helps to release anger, hatred, envy, and distrust. HOLLY brings peace, calmness, and inner joy.

POOL - This switchword improves sharing and teamwork amongst colleagues.

RESTORE - This switchword helps to bring things back to balance. It clears negative feelings between people and restores trust and open-heartedness.

SHUT - This protective switchword helps you to ignore negative words and to be unaffected by destructive criticism. You can use SHUT to end an argument and to stop focusing on any hard words or tension.

THANKS - This master switchword helps to end regret and to bring a close to an argument. THANKS highlights new solutions and shows appreciation.

UBUNTU - This switchword brings participation and co-operation. UBUNTU encourages a feeling of unity, compassion, and generosity.

VINE - This Bach flower remedy brings compassion and improved communication to those who are controlling and domineering.

WATER VIOLET - Another Bach flower remedy switchword. WATER VIOLET softens those who are egotistical and feel that they are superior to others. Use this switchword to help those people to become graceful and compassionate.

Creating a Sigil to clear office politics

To begin creating your sigil, write out a positive statement that reflects your specific desire. It should be in the present tense, so starting with I AM helps. It should only use positive words. Remember, you can use the sigil that I have created below, but it would be far more powerful to create your sigil. Your sigil weaves your focused intention into the sigil, making the sigil send a direct message of your intent to your subconscious.

An example would be -

MY WORK ENVIRONMENT IS POSITIVE AND SUPPORTIVE. I AM VALUED, RESPECTED AND APPRECIATED

Remove all vowels

MYWRKNVRNMNTSPSTVNDSPPRTVMVLDRSPCTDNDPP RCTD

Remove any duplicated letters

MYWRKNTSVDPLC

Draw a sigil using the shapes of the remaining letters. Below is an example of a sigil using the above phrase. You can use this sigil, either as it is, or as inspiration. Remembering that it is so much more powerful for you to create your own sigil.

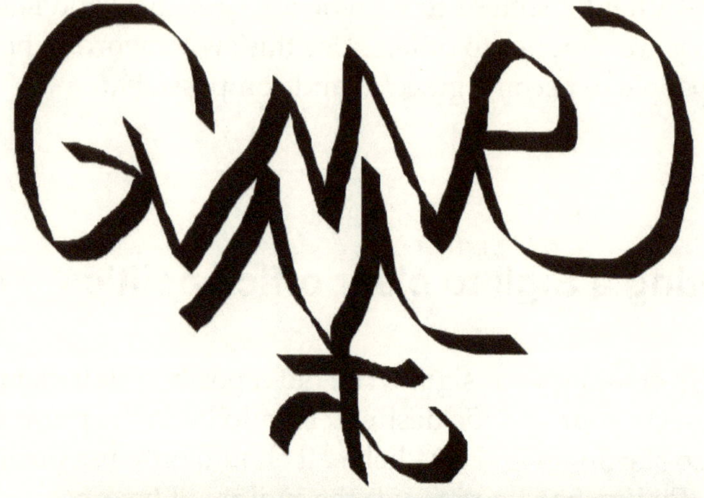

Creating your Energy Circle to clear office politics

Here is an example of an Energy Circle created to remove office politics. To this I would add a drop or two of Clove Oil.

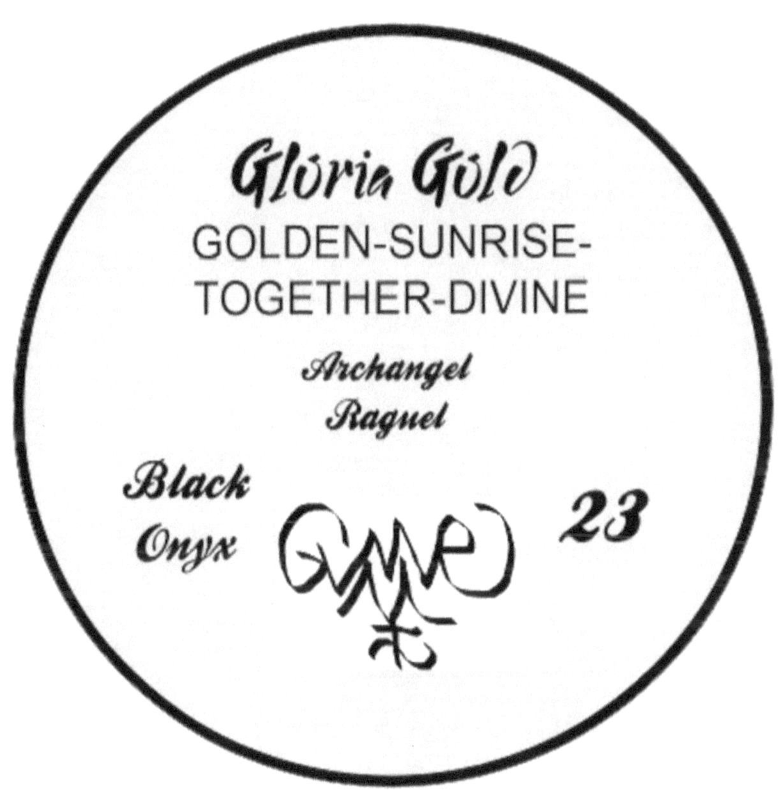

Vibrational Energy for successful Public Speaking

The fear of public speaking, or even speaking up in a meeting can significantly limit your career success. You may have so much value to share, and this fear holds you back. Vibrational energy can help you by increasing your confidence, bringing clarity of mind, giving you courage and determination, and so much more.

Clarifying your request

What types of public speaking would help you to be more successful in your career?

When you picture yourself speaking successfully, how will this feel emotionally, physically and mentally?

How would you like to feel when preparing your talk?

How would you like people to respond to you in this environment?

How would you like to respond to a difficult question?

How would you like to feel after your talk?

Is there anything else that will help you to clarify your desire?

If any of these answers make you feel uncomfortable, work through that, or adjust the question and your response, until you have an unmistakable, joyful feeling when you think about receiving this promotion.

Write your clear desire down, and you can add, 'this or better now comes to me.'

Use this statement and joyful feeling when selecting and working with the energy tools that follow.

Essential Oils for successful public speaking

Cypress - This woody, herbaceous oil helps to release emotions so that you feel calm when public speaking. Did you know that Cupids' arrow is made of Cypress? Imagine shooting love arrows to everyone you're talking to!

Frankincense - Oil of the Gods, this woody, earthy scented oil helps with depression, anxiety, strength, good luck, and self-confidence.

Patchouli - This earthy oil is grounding and calming. It blends well with other oils to create a heady perfume that brings confidence.

Vanilla Absolute - the calming vanilla extract (not quite an essential oil) is wonderfully calming and uplifting.

The following herbs help to increase your confidence - Allspice, Black Pepper, Borage, Cinnamon, Dragon's Blood, Frankincense, Galangal, Geranium, Masterwort, Ragweed, Sweet Pea, Tea, Thyme, Tonka, Wahoo and Yarrow.

Crystals and Gemstones for successful public speaking

Sapphire - Keep this crystal in your pocket, and it will help you to express your thoughts with confidence.

Blue Lace Agate - This comforting stone helps to clear the throat chakra so that you can speak to a crowd. Blue Lace Agate promotes positivity and authenticity. You will feel confident sharing your truth. With this stone, your words will be insightful and articulate.

Numbers for successful public speaking

Number One boosts confidence and gives a sense of leadership in your field. Vibrating at one can help you to come across as an expert on the topic. Number one also makes you more comfortable standing at the podium on your own, facing the crowd.

Colors for successful public speaking

Yellow - The sunshine positivity of yellow brings confidence and warms people to you. Yellow is the color of the solar plexus chakra and helps you to feel confident and empowered. Yellow vibrates at the level of knowledge, inspiration, intellect, and confidence.

Red - The energy of red brings courage and vitality. Red is the color of the root chakra and can help you to feel stable and rooted. Red is also the color of competition and can help you to be a winner at the podium.

Blue is the color of the throat chakra. When this chakra is bright and balanced, you will be able to express yourself clearly and honestly. Blue opens up communication and can help your words to be well received and easily understood.

Angels and Deities for successful public speaking

Archangel Gabriel - This Archangel is the messenger angel. Gabriel will help you to express your message with clarity and with love. Call on this Archangel for help in any area of communication, from writing to marketing and public speaking.

Switchwords for successful public speaking

UP PRAISE - Brings confidence and boosts self-esteem

AIM - This switchword reminds you of the goal and motivates you to move confidently towards it.

ANCHOR - increases confidence and helps you to feel grounded and stable. Attract support & security.

 ASPEN ROCK ROSE MIMULUS - This SWP releases fear, shyness, and trauma, and brings confidence, courage, and strength. This phrase helps you to move forward like a lion.

FAVORITE - Increases admiration from others, and helps you to come across as special and unique.

HUM - This seed mantra for throat chakra brings communication, creativity, truthfulness, integrity, expression. HUM is excellent support when public speaking.

LARCH - This Bach flower remedy raises self-confidence and self-esteem. LARCH will help you to attract opportunities, growth, and success. LARCH releases old fears so that you can embrace new tasks and experiences.

MIMULUS - Another Bach Flower Remedy, MIMULUS helps you to release just about every fear, including the fear of facing a crowd. Gives you the courage to overcome your fears.

SHINE - This powerful switchword removes all negativity. SWITCH helps you to make a positive impression, bringing out your brilliance. SWITCH radiates light and removes all darkness.

SPARKLE - This switchword brings in joy, happiness, liveliness, and excitement. SPARKLE helps you to stand out, and to perform well on stage.

TIGER EYE - This golden gemstone release fear and anxiety. TIGER EYE clears the solar plexus chakra and activates vitality, will power and good luck.

Creating a Sigil for successful public speaking

To begin creating your sigil, write out a positive statement that reflects your specific desire. It should be in the present tense, so starting with I AM helps. It should only use positive words. Remember, you can use the sigil that I have created below, but it would be far more powerful to create your sigil. Your sigil weaves your focused intention into the sigil, making the sigil send a direct message of your intent to your subconscious.

An example would be -

I EASILY AND CONFIDENTLY EXPRESS MYSELF

Remove all vowels

SLYNDCNFDNTLYXPRSSMYSLF

Remove any duplicated letters

SLYNDCFTXPRM

Draw a sigil using the shapes of the remaining letters. Below is an example of a sigil using the above phrase. You can use this sigil, either as it is, or as inspiration. Remembering that it is so much more powerful for you to create your own sigil.

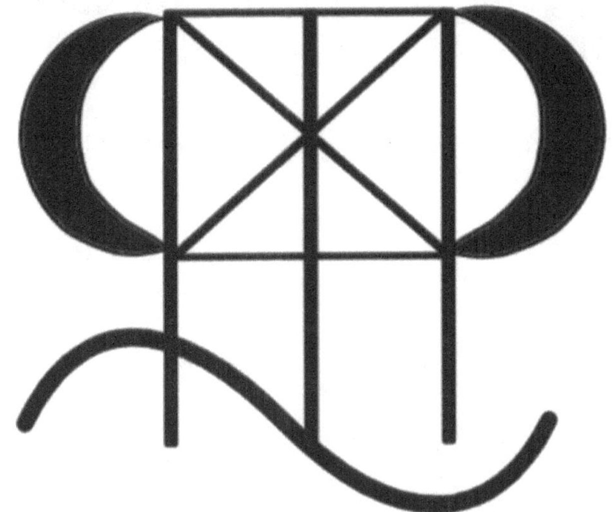

Creating your Energy Circle for successful public speaking

Here is an example of an Energy Circle created to support you when speaking in public.

I would also add a drop or two of patchouli oil to my energy circle.

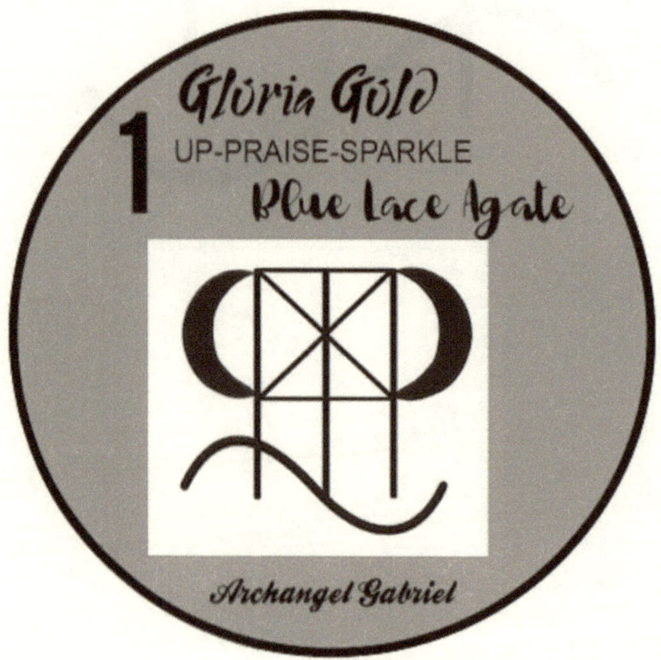

Dearests, I do hope that you have gained value from this book of vibrational energies. May you live your life at the highest vibration, quickly noticing when low energy takes hold, and using your tools to lift yourself up, where good things can easily flow to your matching vibration.

Blessings of joy, love, ease and grace, always.

Much Love,

Gloria Gold

Dearest reader, if you find value in this book, I would SO appreciate a review on Amazon Kindle, so that my book can reach and impact more readers. Thank you! Here's the link: https://www.amazon.com/kindle/dp/B07ZMZDR5Q/ref=r dr_kindle_ext_eos_detail

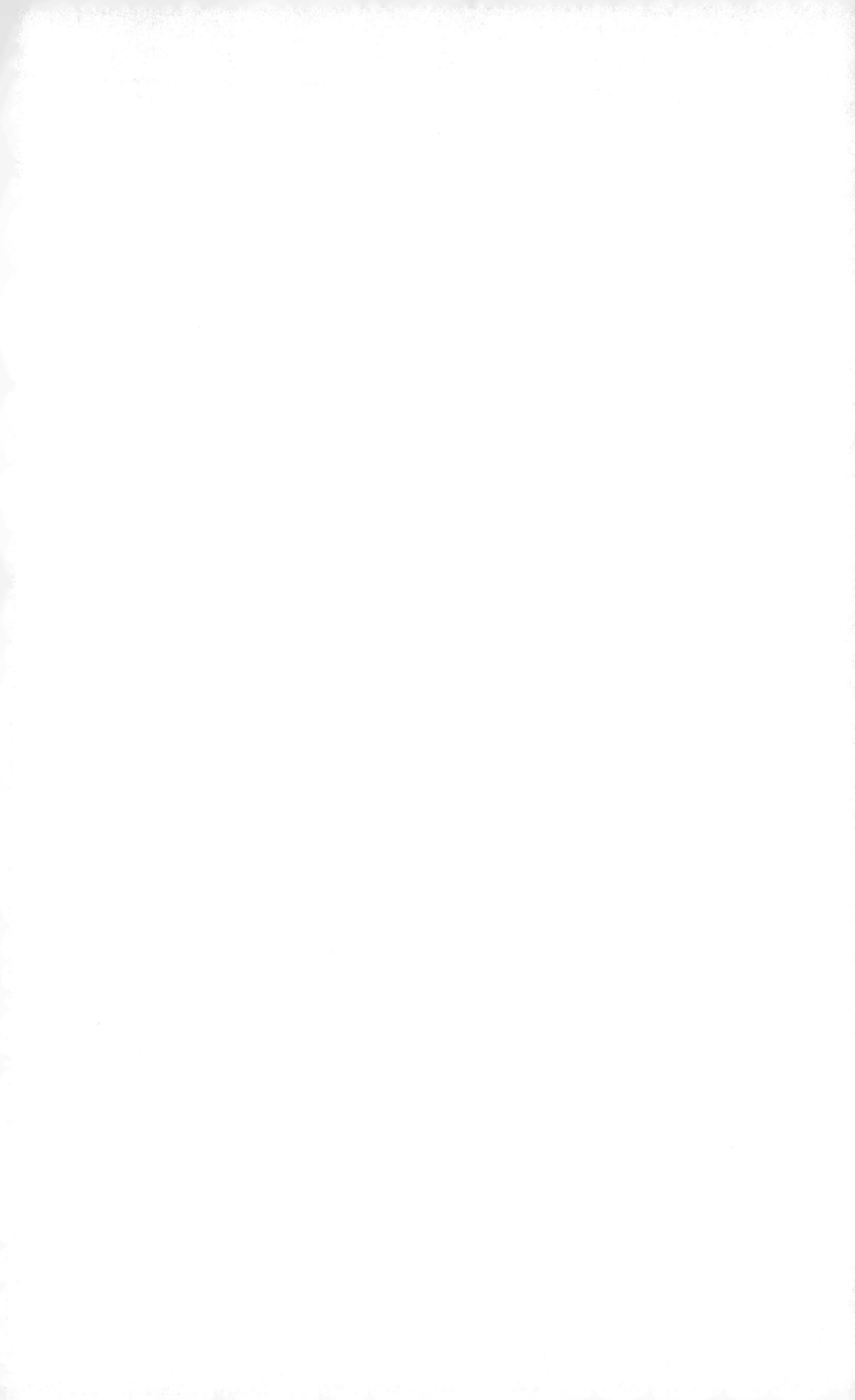